SETTING PRIORITIES FOR HEALTH TECHNOLOGY ASSESSMENT

A MODEL PROCESS

Molla S. Donaldson and Harold C. Sox, Jr., Editors

Committee on Priorities for Assessment and Reassessment
of Health Care Technologies
Institute of Medicine

NATIONAL ACADEMY PRESS
Washington, D.C. 1992

NOTICE: The project that is the subject of this report was approved by the Governing Board of the National Research Council, whose members are drawn from the councils of the National Academy of Sciences, the National Academy of Engineering, and the Institute of Medicine. The members of the committee responsible for this report were chosen for their special competences and with regard for appropriate balance.

This report has been reviewed by a group other than the authors according to procedures approved by a Report Review Committee consisting of members of the National Academy of Sciences, the National Academy of Engineering, and the Institute of Medicine.

The Institute of Medicine was chartered in 1970 by the National Academy of Sciences to enlist distinguished members of the appropriate professions in the examination of policy matters pertaining to the health of the public. In this, the Institute acts under both the Academy's 1863 congressional charter responsibility to be an adviser to the federal government and its own initiative in identifying issues of medical care, research, and education.

Support for this project was provided by the Agency for Health Care Policy and Research and the National Research Council.

Library of Congress Catalog Card No. 92-80702
International Standard Book Number 0-309-04696-3
Additional copies of this report are available from:
National Academy Press
2101 Constitution Avenue, NW
Washington, DC 20418

S-556
Printed in the United States of America

The serpent has been a symbol of long life, healing, and knowledge among almost all cultures and religions since the beginning of recorded history. The image adopted as a logotype by the Institute of Medicine is based on a relief carving from ancient Greece, now held by the Staatlichemuseen in Berlin.

COMMITTEE ON PRIORITIES FOR ASSESSMENT AND REASSESSMENT OF HEALTH CARE TECHNOLOGIES

HAROLD C. SOX, JR. (Chair), Professor and Chair, Department of Medicine, Dartmouth-Hitchcock Medical Center, Lebanon, New Hampshire
ROBERT A. BERENSON, Medical Director, National Capital Preferred Provider Organization and Practitioner in Internal Medicine, Washington, D.C.
PETER BOUXSEIN, Deputy Executive Vice President, American College of Physicians, Philadelphia, Pennsylvania
GLENNA M. CROOKS, Executive Director, Merck and Company, Rahway, New Jersey
B. KRISTINE JOHNSON, Vice President and General Manager, Tachyarrhythmia Division, Medtronic, Inc., Minneapolis, Minnesota
BRYAN R. LUCE, Director, Battelle Medical Technology Assessment and Policy (MEDTAP) Research Center, Washington, D.C.
CHARLES E. PHELPS,[*] Professor and Chair, Department of Community and Preventive Medicine, and Professor, Political Science and Economics, University of Rochester, Rochester, New York
RUTH B. PURTILO, Professor of Clinical Ethics, Center for Health Policy and Ethics, Creighton University, Omaha, Nebraska
MICHAEL F. ROIZEN, Professor and Chair, Department of Anesthesia and Critical Care, and Professor, Department of Internal Medicine, University of Chicago, Chicago, Illinois
CARY S. SENNETT, Medical Director and Director, Clinical Quality Management, AEtna Life and Casualty, Hartford, Connecticut
GEORGE F. SHELDON, Professor and Chair, Department of Surgery, University of North Carolina at Chapel Hill
CATHY SULZBERGER, Chevy Chase, Maryland
GAIL L. WARDEN,[*] President and Chief Executive Officer, Henry Ford Health System, Detroit, Michigan

STUDY STAFF

Division of Health Care Services
KARL D. YORDY, Director
KATHLEEN N. LOHR, Deputy Director
MOLLA S. DONALDSON, Study Director
THERESA H. NALLY, Senior Secretary

---

[*] Member, Institute of Medicine

Acknowledgments

As in any effort of this kind, thanks are due to many people who assisted the committee. Several made presentations at its meetings and reflected on its work. They included Richard Goldbloom of the Canadian Task Force on the Periodic Examination; Thomas Holohan, director of the Office of Technology Assessment at the Agency for Health Care Policy and Research (AHCPR); J. Sanford Schwartz at the Leonard Davis Institute of Health Economics, University of Pennsylvania; and Steven Thacker of the Centers for Disease Control.

As the committee developed its model, it sought and received valuable additional advice, especially on the feasibility of the model, from Clyde Behney at the Office of Technology Assessment, David Eddy of Duke University, Steven Thacker of the Centers for Disease Control, Seymour Perry of the Program on Technology and Health Care at Georgetown University, Linda Johnson White of the Clinical Assessment and Efficacy Program of the American College of Physicians, and representatives of the American Managed Care Review Association, Blue Cross and Blue Shield Association, Group Health Association, the Health Industry Manufacturers Association, the Health Insurance Association of America, and Prudential Insurance Company of America. Kathleen Buto, director of the Bureau of Policy Development of the Health Care Financing Administration, and Michael Hash, senior staff associate for the Subcommittee on Health and the Environment, House Committee on Energy and Commerce, also provided helpful insight on the federal role in technology assessment.

Several members of the Institute of Medicine staff critiqued the manuscript. Annetine Gelijns reviewed Chapter 2. Everette James, an IOM visiting scholar, provided many helpful comments on medical technologies. Richard Rettig provided a wealth of background material and historical knowledge and critiqued Chapter 1. Michael Stoto critiqued an early draft of the quantitative model. Kathleen Lohr not only reviewed the manuscript but helped to solve many quandaries throughout the study—we are particularly appreciative of her efforts. We are also indebted to the staff efforts of Leah Mazade for her skillful editorial review, to Nina Spruill, financial analyst, and to John Devereux and Donna Thompson for their help in preparing the manuscript. Karl Yordy, director of the Division of Health Care Services, provided counsel during the study.

Two other individuals deserve special mention. At Dartmouth-Hitchcock Medical Center, Ray Kulite of MHMH Productions produced a briefing videotape for the committee. Mary Kiernan, executive secretary to Dr. Sox, was unfailingly helpful and gracious.

Finally, financial support for this study was provided by the U.S. Public Health Service, Department of Health and Human Services, and the National Research Council. The committee would like to acknowledge the valuable assistance of Steven Hotta, in AHCPR's Office of Health Technology Assessment, who acted as the study's project officer.

Contents

PREFACE	xiii
SUMMARY	1
Rationale,	1
Methods of Priority Setting,	2
Guiding Principles,	3
The Process Proposed by the IOM Committee,	4
Steps in the Process,	4
Seven Criteria,	5
Reassessment,	5
The Priority-Setting Cycle,	5
Human Resources Required to Implement the Process,	6
Publicly Available Products,	6
Topics for Which There Is Insufficient Evidence to Conduct an Assessment Based on Review of the Literature,	6
Recommendations,	6
Recommendation 1,	8
Recommendation 2,	8
Recommendation 3,	9
Recommendation 4,	9
Recommendation 5,	10
Recommendation 6,	11
Recommendation 7,	11
Recommendation 8,	12

Recommendation 9,	12
Recommendation 10,	12
Recommendation 11,	13
Adoption of the IOM's Priority-Setting Process by Other Organizations,	13
Technology Assessment and Clinical Practice Guidelines,	14
Potential Problems with the Priority-Setting Process,	15
Concluding Remarks,	15

1 TECHNOLOGY ASSESSMENT AND THE NEED FOR PRIORITY SETTING — 17

Evolution of Technology Assessment Toward Outcomes, Effectiveness, and Appropriateness Research,	18
The Effectiveness Initiative and Establishment of the Agency for Health Care Policy and Research,	20
The Office of Health Technology Assessment,	20
Origin of the IOM Study,	21
Previous Pilot Study of Preliminary Model,	21
Study Methods,	22
Definitions,	23
Medical Technology,	23
Technology Assessment,	23
Reassessment,	25
Report Structure,	26
Summary,	26
Appendix: The Agency for Health Care Policy and Research,	26
Center for Medical Effectiveness Research,	27
Office of the Forum for Quality and Effectiveness in Health Care,	27
Office of Science and Data Development,	27
Center for General Health Services Extramural Research and the Division of Technology and Quality Assessment,	28
Office of Health Technology Assessment,	28

2 METHODS FOR PRIORITY SETTING — 31

Priority-Setting Processes Used by Organizations,	32
Example 1: Health Care Financing Administration,	32
Example 2: Private Sector Pharmaceutical Industry,	33
Example 3: Health Care Provider Organizations,	35
Example 4: Institute of Medicine/Council on Health Care Technology Pilot Study,	36
Example 5: Food and Drug Administration,	37
Quantitative Models for Setting Priorities,	38

		Example 6: Technology Assessment Priority-Setting System,	38
		Example 7: The Phelps-Parente Model,	38
		Setting Priorities for Spending on Health Services,	39
		Example 8: Oregon Basic Health Services Act,	39
		Discussion,	41
		Reactive and Implicit Processes,	41
		Analytic Models,	43
		Need for a Comprehensive, Proactive Process for Priority Setting,	44
		Summary,	44
		Appendix: Medicare Coverage Decision Making,	45
3	**GUIDING PRINCIPLES**		50
		Building a Model Process for Setting Priorities,	50
		Process Building for OHTA,	51
		The Process Must Reflect the Mission of OHTA,	51
		The Product of the Process Should Be Consistent with the Needs of Users,	53
		The Process Must Be Efficient,	54
		The Process Must Be Sensitive to the Environment in Which OHTA Operates,	55
		Summary,	56
4	**RECOMMENDATIONS FOR A PRIORITY-SETTING PROCESS**		57
		Preview of the Quantitative Model,	59
		Elements of the Proposed Priority-Setting Process,	60
		Step 1. Selecting and Weighting Criteria Used to Establish Priorities,	60
		Step 2. Identifying Candidate Conditions and Technologies,	61
		Step 3. Winnowing the List of Candidate Conditions and Technologies,	62
		Step 4. Data Gathering,	62
		Step 5. Creating Criterion Scores,	62
		Step 6. Computing Priority Scores,	63
		Step 7. Review by AHCPR National Advisory Council,	64
		Details of the Proposed Priority-Setting Process,	64
		Step 1. Selecting and Weighting the Criteria Used to Establish Priority Scores,	64
		Step 2. Identifying Candidate Conditions and Technologies,	66
		Step 3. Winnowing the List of Candidate Conditions and Technologies,	66
		Step 4. Data Gathering,	68

	Step 5. Creating Criterion Scores,	69
	Step 6. Computing Priority Scores,	83
	Step 7. Review by AHCPR National Advisory Council,	87
	Reassessment,	88
	Role of Reassessment in the Complete Assessment Program,	88
	Methods of Identifying Candidates for Reassessment,	90
	Final Steps After Establishing Priority for Reassessment,	94
	Summary,	94
Appendix 4.1:	Winnowing Processes,	95
	Intensity Rankings by Nominating Persons and Organizations,	95
	Preliminary Ranking Processes,	97
	Panel-Based Preliminary Weighting,	98
	Comment,	99
Appendix 4.2:	Methodologic Issues,	100
	Properties of Logarithms,	101
	Application to the IOM Model,	102
5	**IMPLEMENTATION ISSUES**	**103**
	The Priority-Setting Cycle,	103
	Setting Criterion Weights,	104
	Resources Needed to Implement the Process,	105
	Technology Assessment Program Staff Requirements,	105
	Priority-Setting Panel,	106
	Implementation Considerations for OHTA and Other Organizations,	108
	Validity and Reliability,	108
	Criteria,	109
	Availability of Data to Generate Criterion Scores,	110
	Publicly Available Products,	110
	When the Scientific Evidence Is Insufficient for Assessment,	111
	Interim Statements,	112
	Modeling,	112
	Summary,	113
6	**RECOMMENDATIONS AND CONCLUSIONS**	**115**
	Review of the Committee's Rationale and Recommendations,	115
	Recommendations,	116
	Review of Steps and Issues in Implementation,	122
	Steps in a Priority-Setting Process,	122
	Resources for Implementation,	123
	The Priority-Setting Cycle,	124
	Publicly Available Products,	124

	Topics with Insufficient Evidence for Assessment Based on Review of the Literature,	124
	Adoption of the IOM'S Priority-Setting Process by Other Organizations,	125
	Technology Assessment and Clinical Practice Guidelines,	127
	Potential Problems with the Priority-Setting Process,	127
	Will a Numerical Priority Score Lead to Unrealistic Inferences About Priority?	128
	Does Codifying an Idealized Process Lead to Inflexibility?	128
	Will There Be a Bias Toward Choosing Topics That Are Quantifiable?	128
	Conclusion,	129
	REFERENCES	131
APPENDIX A:	**PILOT TEST OF THE IOM MODEL**	136
	Methods,	137
	Topics and Data for Priority Setting,	137
	Criteria,	137
	Criterion Weighting,	138
	Criterion Scoring,	138
	Results,	139
	Feasibility,	139
	Improvements in the Model,	139
	Comparison of Convened and Mailed Methods,	139
	Priority Scores,	141
	Implications of the Pilot Tests for the IOM Model,	143
	Criterion Scores,	144
APPENDIX B:	**ABBREVIATIONS**	146

Preface

The immediate objective of this report is to provide a government agency with a method for deciding which health care technologies it should evaluate. The origin of the task is the 1989 legislation that authorized the creation of the Agency for Health Care Policy and Research. The legislation called upon the new agency to promote health care technology assessment by, among other means, deciding which technologies are the most important to evaluate. The agency asked the Institute of Medicine to study methods for setting priorities and to advise its Office of Health Technology Assessment.

The problem of deciding which health technologies to evaluate is a new problem, and it is urgent. Health technology assessment itself is a new field. It came to fruition during the 1980s, when new health technologies proliferated alongside steadily increasing health care costs. Many experts blamed physicians for indiscriminately using these technologies. The real problem was our failure to do the research that can teach us how to be discriminating. Directing tests and treatments at those who can benefit the most is the unmet challenge. Technology assessment can help to solve this problem by discovering the answer to the question, "What works in the practice of medicine?" The answer can often be found by applying rigorous epidemiologic thinking to the published literature. The problem is that there are many clinical problems and technologies to be evaluated, many months of work required to study one problem, and relatively few clinicians with highly developed analytic skills. Therefore, institutions must set priorities.

When the Agency for Health Care Policy and Research asked for advice, the Institute of Medicine convened a study group. Our committee's first task was to learn how organizations set priorities. We found that there is little published literature on priority setting in the health field. Unfettered by tradition, we sought a method that would satisfy several criteria that we felt should be important to any public agency. First, the method should provide opportunities for the public to express its values. Second, the method should be explicit, so that people can trace backwards from results to inputs and so satisfy themselves that the process was fair. Third, priority for assessment should reflect the potential benefit to the public from doing an assessment.

Will this report have a broad readership? We certainly hope so. The Institute of Medicine gave us a broad mandate: satisfy the needs of the agency but keep in mind the needs of other organizations that do technology assessment. We therefore tried to develop a generally applicable method for setting priorities. We hope that other organizations will find this priority-setting method to be useful. Some organizations may find the entire method to their liking; others will find some elements of it attractive and will reject others. As authors, we will be quite pleased if we can engage the reader's interest in a problem that we found challenging and important.

Harold C. Sox, Jr., M.D.

Chair, Committee on Priorities for Assessmentand Reassessment of Health Care Technologies

SETTING PRIORITIES FOR HEALTH TECHNOLOGY ASSESSMENT

A MODEL PROCESS

Summary

The Institute of Medicine (IOM) Committee on Priorities for Assessment and Reassessment of Health Care Technologies was charged to propose a process for setting priorities for technology assessment in the Office of Health Technology Assessment (OHTA) of the Agency for Health Care Policy and Research (AHCPR) and in other assessment organizations. (AHCPR is part of the U.S. Public Health Service.) In responding to this charge, the committee organized its work and this report at three levels of specification: general principles, a proposed process, and information about how to implement the process in OHTA and other organizations that conduct health technology assessment.

This summary reviews the main points of the report: the rationale for the process developed by the committee, the committee's 11 recommendations, seven steps needed to implement the proposed process, anticipated resources and periodicity of the process, and implementation issues that require consideration. Further, it examines how the proposed priority-setting process might be used or adapted by other organizations and for purposes other than technology assessment.

RATIONALE

Clinicians, payers, and policymakers turn to technology assessment to help provide better information for clinical decision making, to guide coverage decisions, and to set national health policy. Technology assessment can play a valuable role in the entire process of improvement of health and health care. For example, an assessment may show that the data needed for a complete evaluation of a technology are not available. This finding may serve as an impetus to initiate research to supply the missing information. Similarly, an assessment may lead to changes in practice norms when it yields a conclusion that differs from common clinical behavior.

Yet efficient use of resources for technology assessment requires a systematic priority-setting process. In the legislation establishing AHCPR, the IOM was asked to develop a process and criteria for setting priorities for health care technology assessment and reassessment to assist OHTA in its expanded role within that agency. The establishment of AHCPR itself can be seen as recognition of the need to look systematically at the value of health care services in improving health. This kind of assessment uses measures of effectiveness as a means of better understanding the appropriate use of new and established technologies; the expansion of the role of OHTA to develop a comprehensive process to guide this work is consistent with that goal. Such a process should also be of value to other organizations that, notwithstanding their different goals, must develop priorities for the use of limited assessment resources.

METHODS OF PRIORITY SETTING

The committee described several examples of priority setting from a number of different organizations or groups: (1) the Health Care Financing Administration; (2) a research-intensive pharmaceutical company; (3) the Clinical Efficacy and Assessment Program of the American College of Physicians and the Diagnostic and Therapeutic Technology Assessment Program of the American Medical Association; (4) the priority-setting process used by the IOM's Council on Health Care Technology in its 1990 pilot study; (5) the Food and Drug Administration; two examples of quantitative models of priority setting—(6) David Eddy's Technology Assessment Priority-Setting System and (7) the Phelps and Parente model; and (8) the process developed under the Oregon Basic Health Services Act to set priorities for Medicaid spending.

The committee drew on these examples to derive a set of principles for developing a process for OHTA to use in setting priorities. Although individual assessment organizations may have various goals in assessment, the public as a whole has an interest in the effects and use of medical technologies. Public agencies need a comprehensive, proactive process of public input to ensure that the technology assessment provides the greatest gain to the health of the public. In addition, priority setting must be accountable to the public. It cannot be private, implicit, or internal to the organization, and it must include a process that is open, fair, and credible to discriminate among the array of possible technologies that it might assess or reassess.

There are a number of benefits to be derived from the use of analytic models—they structure thinking, use what data are available, open the process to review and accountability, and are amenable to examination and adjustment of both the results and the methodology. Such models move the technology assessment process closer to a realization of its potential for strengthening the scientific basis for decision making. The use of analytic models, however, is more complex and requires more resources (at least initially) and expertise than an implicit process that simply reacts to requests for technology assessment. The committee concluded that any analytic model must include a process to review its product, and a way to include issues of equity, as well as unusual ethical and legal dimensions presented by health care technologies. Nevertheless, priority rankings established by means of an analytic model should be understood as inputs to a final decision process, not the final product of the process itself.

GUIDING PRINCIPLES

The committee formulated several general principles to direct its development of a priority-setting process. The first such principle is that any priority-setting process for technology assessment must be consistent with the mission of the organization that uses it. For a public agency, the values of the public that the agency serves need to be incorporated into the priority-setting process. Such a process for OHTA will have to assemble information about the potential of a technology to improve health outcomes, to reduce inappropriate expenditures, to redress inequity among those receiving health care, and to inform special social issues.

Second, the priority-setting process must consider the information needs of users. The process designed for OHTA should, in general, focus on technology assessment for *specific clinical conditions* and on *alternative approaches* to management of those conditions.

Third, the priority-setting process must be efficient so that scarce resources for technology assessment are not needlessly consumed in the process of setting assessment priorities. OHTA should seek broad input at the outset, but it should also have some relatively simple mechanism to identify the important topics. The process should also take advantage of available data or, where data are lacking, of subjective judgments, rather than require the collection of new data.

Finally, the priority-setting process must be sensitive to its political context; it must be—and must appear to be—objective, open, and fair; it must invite input from a variety of interested parties; and it must present the logic of the process clearly and carefully to others.

THE PROCESS PROPOSED BY THE IOM COMMITTEE

Steps in the Process

The committee presents below the description of a process that can be understood as logically deriving from consideration of the issues noted in the above principles. Figure S.1 shows seven elements: (1) selecting and weighting criteria for establishing priorities: (2) eliciting broad input for candidate conditions and technologies; (3) winnowing the number of topics; (4) gathering the data needed to assign a score for each priority-setting

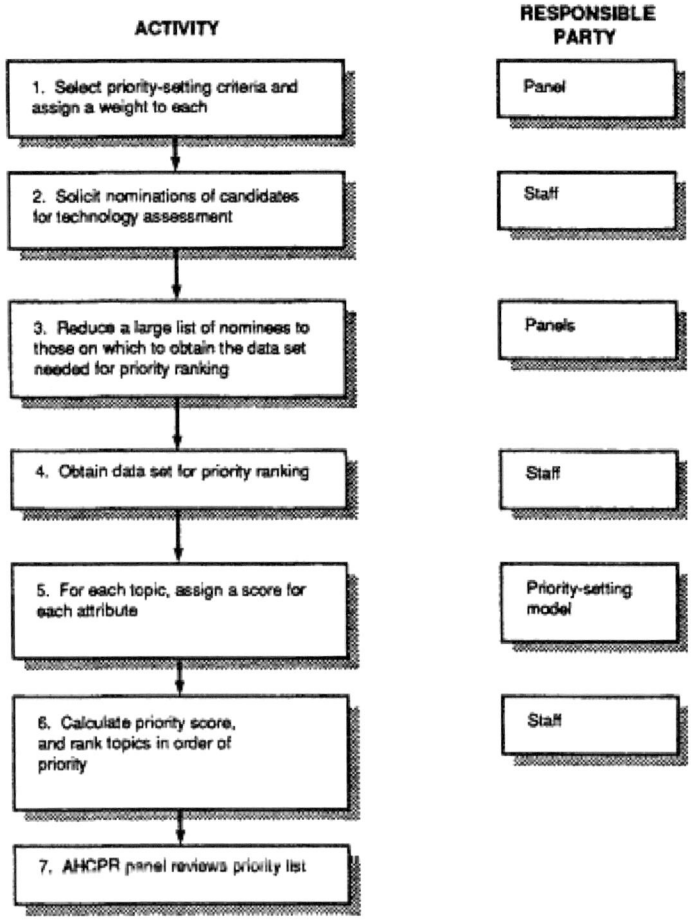

Figure S.1 Overview of the IOM priority-setting process.

criterion for each topic; (5) assigning criterion scores for each topic, using objective data for some criteria and a rating scale anchored by low- and high-priority topics for subjective criteria; (6) calculating priority scores for each condition or technology and ranking the topics in order of priority; and (7) requesting review by the AHCPR National Advisory Council.

Seven Criteria

The committee recommended and defined seven priority-setting criteria and explained how to assign scores for each of them. Three of the criteria are objective—prevalence, cost, and clinical practice variations; they are scored using quantitative data to the extent possible. Four of the criteria are subjective—burden of illness, and the likelihood that the results of the assessment will affect patient outcomes, costs, and ethical, legal, and social issues; these criteria are scored according to ratings on a scale from 1 to 5.

Reassessment

Certain aspects of priority setting apply only to reassessment of previously assessed technologies: these include recognizing events that trigger reassessment (e.g., changes in the nature of the condition, in knowledge, or in clinical practice); the need to track information related to previous assessments; and the obligation to update a previous assessment as a fiduciary responsibility and to preserve the credibility of the assessing organization.

Because the committee believes that OHTA has a special obligation to consider previously assessed topics as candidates for reassessment, it also believes that the agency should maintain a process for monitoring the published literature on previously assessed topics and should place candidates for reassessment on the same competitive footing in the priority-setting process as candidates for first-time assessment.

The Priority-Setting Cycle

The committee envisions priority setting as occurring in a cycle. The panel (see below) sets criterion weights approximately every 5 years. The priority-setting cycle itself repeats at least once every 3 years and leads to a rank-ordered list of conditions and technologies. The priority-setting cycle begins and ends with involvement of persons and institutions outside the federal government. At the beginning, OHTA asks a broad range of persons and institutions to nominate conditions and technologies that they wish to have assessed. OHTA staff collect the data required to set objective crite rion scores and convene panels to assign criterion scores to each condition or technology.

Human Resources Required to Implement the Process

A broadly representative panel would set criterion weights, reduce the list of nominations of conditions or technologies, and assign criterion scores to each of these topics. Subpanels might be required to divide the workload; the subpanels would need to be separately constituted to assign subjective or objective criterion scores. The subpanel(s) assigning *subjective* criterion scores would be composed of individuals with the same range of perspectives as the full panel. The subpanel(s) assigning *objective* criterion scores would require experts in epidemiology and health statistics to review the data collected by OHTA staff and to develop estimates when necessary.

Publicly Available Products

The committee envisions two products of the priority-setting process that would be publicly available: a list of the priority-ranked technologies and the data base used to construct the list. Both would contribute to a priority-setting document published by OHTA. Each highly ranked technology should also be accompanied by a discussion of the features that contributed to its ranking, the data sources used, the level of confidence the panels assigned to the data, and any strongly held minority views.

Topics for Which There is Insufficient Evidence to Conduct an Assessment Based on Review of the Literature

OHTA should adopt methods that will enable it to conduct preliminary assessments even when there is not yet adequate evidence on which to base a strong clinical policy recommendation. For topics that are of high priority for assessment but for which there is insufficient evidence, the committee particularly recommends using decision analysis as a way to identify which missing evidence is most important for decision making. These results can then be used as input to the development of an agenda for empirical research sponsored by AHCPR. This concept of linking priority setting, assessment of the evidence, and a research agenda is very important to the future of technology assessment and of evidence-based medical practice.

RECOMMENDATIONS

The committee's recommendations are listed in Table S.1 and are described briefly below.

Table S.1 Recommendations

RECOMMENDATION 1
OHTA should adopt a systematic process to assist decision making about which medical conditions and technologies it should assess or reassess. The process should involve a broad spectrum of interested parties and should be open to public view, resistant to control by special interests, and clearly understandable.

RECOMMENDATION 2
OHTA technology assessment, whenever feasible, should focus on a clinical problem (e.g., diagnosis of coronary artery disease) rather than on a technology per se (e.g., exercise thallium radionuclide scan). Similarly, priority setting should address clinical conditions.

RECOMMENDATION 3
OHTA technology assessments should compare the alternative technologies for managing a clinical condition. Similarly, the priority-setting process should include alternative technologies for managing a clinical condition.

RECOMMENDATION 4
OHTA should identify criteria that best characterize a topic's importance as a candidate for assessment. The committee recommends the following *objective criteria*:
- prevalence of the specific condition;
- unit cost of the technologies commonly used to manage the condition (or the unit cost of a technology and its alternatives); and
- variation in the rate of use of a technology for managing the condition (or variations in the rates of use of the technology and its alternatives).

The committee also recommends the following *subjective criteria*:
- burden of illness imposed by the clinical condition;
- potential of the results of the assessment to change health outcomes;
- potential of the results of the assessment to change costs; and
- potential of the results of the assessment to inform ethical, legal, or social issues.

RECOMMENDATION 5
OHTA should use an explicit process to determine a candidate topic's priority ranking. In the ranking process, the criteria that are important in deciding whether to do an assessment determine a topic's priority rank.

RECOMMENDATION 6
The committee recommends a specific quantitative method to calculate a priority score for each candidate topic using the following formula:

$$\text{Priority Score} = W_1 \ln S_1 + W_2 \ln S_2 + \ldots + W_7 \ln S_7$$

where W is the criterion weight, S is the criterion score, and ln is the natural logarithm of the criterion scores.
A panel of people from a broad spectrum of interests should set the criterion weights.

RECOMMENDATION 7
OHTA should actively solicit nominations of topics to be considered for assessment. The solicitation should include payers, health professionals and their representative organizations, manufacturers of medical products, business, labor, government agencies, and consumers of health care.

RECOMMENDATION 8
OHTA should develop a structured procedure for reducing the number of nominations.

RECOMMENDATION 9
OHTA should consider all previously assessed topics as candidates for reassessment.

RECOMMENDATION 10
OHTA should maintain a data base on each topic that has been previously assessed and should catalog information pertaining to the topic.

RECOMMENDATION 11
OHTA should set priorities among topics for reassessment at the same time and on the same footing that it sets priorities for first-time assessment. That is, the committee recommends that OHTA create one rank-ordered list that contains both topics for reassessment and topics for first-time assessment.

Recommendation 1

OHTA should adopt a systematic process to assist decision making about which medical conditions and technologies it should assess or reassess. The process should involve a broad spectrum of interested parties and should be open to public view, resistant to control by special interests, and clearly understandable.

The process proposed by the committee would be conducted in two phases —the setting of weights for criteria, which is performed approximately every 5 years, and the rest of the priority-setting process, which is performed approximately every 3 years.

Recommendation 2

OHTA technology assessment, whenever feasible, should focus on a clinical problem (e.g., diagnosis of coronary artery disease) rather than on a technology per se (e.g., exercise thallium radionuclide scan). Similarly, priority setting should address clinical conditions.

Although concern about a new test or treatment often leads to calls for its assessment, whenever possible, a technology should be evaluated within the context of the clinical condition for which it is being used. There are two reasons for proposing this orientation. First, technology assessment should be comparative, implying that it should answer a useful *clinical* question: Which technology should a practitioner use and under what clinical circumstances? Second, a technology can only be evaluated in the context of what it does, which is to help solve a clinical problem.

Recommendation 3

OHTA technology assessments should compare the alternative technologies for managing a clinical condition. Similarly, the priority-setting process should include alternative technologies for managing a clinical condition.

The data required to determine the assessment priority of a clinical condition depend on which technologies are relevant to its management. (For example, the expected cost of managing a condition depends on the costs of the individual technologies that might be used.)

Many parties need information about alternative technologies for managing a condition. For instance, clinicians and patients must choose among alternatives tests and treatments. Third parties, too, are concerned about the marginal effects of a technology—the additional benefits and risks represented by one technology in comparison with another. This recommendation holds true even when a new technology is the first to be applied to a clinical problem: when there are no obvious comparative *technologies*, watchful waiting without therapeutic intervention is always a valid, and important, alternative.

The comparison of technologies should take place on a "level playing field"; that is, the same methods and similar circumstances should be applied to all of the technologies.

Recommendation 4

OHTA should identify criteria that best characterize a topic's importance as a candidate for assessment. The committee recommends the following *objective criteria*:

- prevalence of the specific condition;
- unit cost of the technologies commonly used to manage the condition (or the unit cost of a technology and its alternatives); and
- variation in the rate of use of a technology for managing the condition (or variations in the rates of use of the technology and its alternatives).

Ordinarily, the data required to characterize a candidate topic may be found in the published literature or elsewhere in the public record. *Prevalence* is the number of people with the condition per 1,000 persons in the general population. *Unit cost* is the total direct and induced cost of conventional management for a person with the clinical condition. *Variation in rates of use* across different settings of care is measured by the coefficient of variation. A high coefficient of variation frequently implies a low level of consensus about clinical management.

The committee also recommends the following *subjective criteria*:

- **burden of illness imposed by the clinical condition;**
- **potential of the results of the assessment to change health outcomes;**
- **potential of the results of the assessment to change costs; and**
- **potential of the results of the assessment to inform ethical, legal, or social issues.**

Although objective data may exist with which to characterize a candidate topic, integration of these data often requires a subjective estimate. *Burden of illness*, which is estimated at the level of the patient rather than of society, is the difference between the quality-adjusted life expectancy (QALE) of a patient who has the condition and who receives conventional treatment and the QALE of a person of the same age who does not have the condition. The potential of the results of the assessment to *change health outcomes* is the expected effect of the result of the assessment on health outcomes for patients with the illness. It includes consideration of the findings of the assessment and of the likelihood of policy and administrative changes, clinical practice changes, and patient acceptance. The potential of the results of an assessment to *change costs* is the expected effect of the results of an assessment on the costs of illness for patients with the illness. It includes direct costs to the patient and induced costs.

The committee anticipates that most conditions will be adequately ranked based on the first six criteria listed above. The seventh criterion—the potential of the results of the assessment to *inform ethical, legal, or social issues*—gives the priority-setting panelists the opportunity to take a broad social perspective and to ask whether there is anything that has not been captured in the first six criteria that would alter the priority listing of a particular topic.

Recommendation 5

OHTA should use an explicit process to determine a candidate topic's priority ranking. In the ranking process, the criteria that are important in deciding whether to do an assessment determine a topic's priority rank.

SUMMARY

The committee recommends the use of a process that can be examined, challenged, and adjusted on the basis of tests of its reliability and validity. Use of a quantitative model as part of this process allows assumptions to be explicitly stated and individually assessed; it also permits the use of data, whenever they are available.

Recommendation 6

The committee recommends a specific quantitative method to calculate a priority score for each candidate topic using the following formula:

$$\text{Priority Score} = W_1 \ln S_1 + W_2 \ln S_2 + \ldots + W_7 \ln S_7$$

where W is the criterion weight, S is the criterion score, and ln is the natural logarithm of the criterion scores.

A panel of people from a broad spectrum of interests should set the criterion weights.

In the process proposed by the committee, a broadly based panel would be created to lead the necessary activities. Its first task would be to establish the criterion weights through one of several possible procedures that are detailed in the full report. Once established, these criterion weights remain constant for the entire priority-setting process (i.e., across all candidate topics).

A topic's priority score determines its priority rank. According to the committee's method, each candidate topic receives a criterion score for each of the seven criteria (for example, S_1 might be prevalence expressed as a number per 1,000 persons in the general population). In addition, each criterion has a criterion weight that reflects its importance in determining priorities for technology assessment. (W_1, for example, might be a weight of 2 for prevalence, relative to a burden-of-illness criterion weight of 3.)

Each candidate *topic* has its own combination of criterion scores (S_n) for the seven attributes. The panel noted above (or a subset of its members) reviews data prepared for each topic by OHTA staff and assigns the criterion scores. Objective criterion scores are determined by a subpanel with expertise in clinical epidemiology and statistics. Subjective criterion scores are determined by a broadly representative panel (or subpanel) with expertise in health care.

Recommendation 7

OHTA should actively solicit nominations of topics to be considered for assessment. The solicitation should include payers, health professionals

and their representative organizations, manufacturers of medical products, business, labor, government agencies, and consumers of health care.

The committee judged that a widespread solicitation of topics is crucial to the success of the priority-setting effort. In particular, the solicitation should be broad enough to ensure that important technologies are not omitted inadvertently from consideration and that all important constituencies are included in the process.

Recommendation 8

OHTA should develop a structured procedure for reducing the number of nominations.

The initial number of nominations will almost certainly far exceed staff capacity to collect the data required to assign criterion scores to each topic. Therefore, the committee proposes that a formal procedure be adopted to reduce that initial list to a manageable size—a technique it calls "winnowing." The full report describes three possible methods of winnowing and proposes one for OHTA.

Recommendation 9

OHTA should consider all previously assessed topics as candidates for reassessment.

OHTA has a special obligation as an influential public agency to revisit any previously assessed topics whose recommendations may be based on outdated or now erroneous information. A change in the nature of the condition, expanded professional knowledge, a shift in clinical practice, or publication of a new, conflicting assessment might trigger consideration of a condition and technology for reassessment.

Recommendation 10

OHTA should maintain a data base on each topic that has been previously assessed and should catalog information pertaining to the topic.

A catalog will make it easier for OHTA to know when to consider topics for reassessment and when newly published information is relevant to a topic that has been previously assessed. Information should include descriptions of data, populations, and methods used in the earlier assessment, the impact and controversy generated, and a topic-specific estimated date or interval for considering reassessment.

Recommendation 11

OHTA should set priorities among topics for reassessment at the same time and on the same footing that it sets priorities for first-time assessment. That is, the committee recommends that OHTA create one rank-ordered list that contains both topics for reassessment and topics for first-time assessment.

The process of determining the need for reassessment can be accommodated within a priority-setting process for first-time assessments with the addition of several specific components: (1) a system for tracking previous assessments and events that prompt recognition that a major factor (e.g., a clinical condition or practice, information) has changed relative to the old assessment; (2) evaluation of literature that suggests that reassessment might be needed; (3) a decision by the priority-setting panel that a technology or clinical practice has changed sufficiently to warrant reassessment; and (4) a sensitivity analysis that suggests that the conclusion of an initial assessment might change when a reassessment is conducted.

ADOPTION OF THE IOM'S PRIORITY-SETTING PROCESS BY OTHER ORGANIZATIONS

Many organizations evaluate health technology, although the major categories of such organizations are third-party payers, such as the Health Care Financing Administration (HCFA) and the Blue Cross and Blue Shield Association (BCBSA), and associations that represent physicians, such as the American College of Physicians. The committee developed this proposal for a priority-setting process with the expectation that the process would apply and be useful to these and similar organizations, as well as to OHTA. That expectation is based on the following:

- Although these organizations are part of the private sector, they also constitute a major public resource, both individually and collectively. The more they structure their technology assessment activities, including priority setting, as a public service, the greater the good they will do for their own private purposes and for their mission of public service. By focusing on clinical conditions rather than on individual technologies, their assessments are more likely to compare relevant alternative patient care strategies.
- The argument that priorities for assessment should be determined by several attributes is quite generalizable. An organization that uses only one dimension (e.g., cost, burden of illness) is oversimplifying a very complex matter. The trade-off between cost and effectiveness is one of the most

important questions that physicians and patients must understand and resolve daily in the office or hospital.
- Because the committee's process accommodates the choice of any priority-setting criteria, an organization may choose criteria that serve its own interests. The committee argues, however, that public trust, which sustains any large organization of payers or professionals, requires criteria that are responsive to the public interest, as exemplified by the committee's seven criteria.
- If one accepts the argument that any organization performing health technology assessment, or the officers of that organization who are responsible for the technology assessment, are accountable to the public, at least in very general terms, it would seem to follow that any process of establishing priority rankings should be open, explicit, and understandable.
- The process of soliciting nominations is one element of an ideal process that could be designed to satisfy the needs of a specific organization without compromising the public interest.
- The committee believes that any program of technology assessment must encompass a commitment to reassess topics that have been previously assessed. This commitment must be supported by a program to monitor previously assessed topics for new information that might prompt a reassessment. The rationale for this recommendation is public accountability, but it applies to private interests as well. For example, an organization of physicians should not have a potentially obsolete policy on the public record. Neither should a payer continue to provide or to withhold coverage on the basis of information that may have been superseded by newly published data.

Technology Assessment and Clinical Practice Guidelines

The committee's priority-setting process may also be useful in setting priorities for developing practice guidelines. Clinical practice guidelines, according to another IOM committee's definition, are "systematically developed statements to assist the practitioner and patient in decisions concerning appropriate health care for specific clinical circumstances."

Clinical practice guidelines are one vehicle for disseminating the results of technology assessment, and technology assessment is one method of producing information for a practice guideline. In particular, clinical practice guidelines may use the synthesis of available evidence and projection of outcomes that are a part of technology assessment as a foundation for statements that are clinically useful in individual patient care. Good practice guidelines go one step further, however, to rely on expert consensus to develop practical advice for clinicians in situations not directly addressed by clinical research.

What further distinguishes practice guidelines from technology assessment is the requirement that guidelines very carefully and explicitly describe the thinking that links the evidence (that is, the product of the technology assessment), or the lack of evidence, with the advice. Nonetheless, because technology assessment is so closely related to the development of practice guidelines, the priority-setting process proposed in this report appears to be largely, if not completely, applicable to guidelines development as well.

POTENTIAL PROBLEMS WITH THE PRIORITY-SETTING PROCESS

The report discusses several potential problems with the proposed priority-setting process. For example, will a numerical priority score lead to unrealistic inferences about the precision of the ranks? Does codifying an idealized process lead to inflexibility? Will there be a bias toward choosing topics that are quantifiable? The committee believes that most of these apparent difficulties are the result of misperceptions stemming from the use of a quantitative model to calculate a priority score for an assessment candidate. The great advantages of the model process are that it is explicit, that it contains a representation of the values of society, and that it defines the information-gathering tasks involved in priority setting.

CONCLUDING REMARKS

Although this committee has recommended a specific step-by-step methodology as a priority-setting process, it believes that the four principles noted earlier in this summary are far more important than the specifics of its model. In the case of OHTA, satisfying the first principle will require determining which assessments are most likely to result in improvement in the health of the public, reduction of inappropriate health care expenditures, reduction of inequities in access to effective health care services or of maldistribution across equally needy populations, and the informing of other ethical, legal, and social issues.

OHTA and other organizations may wish to modify some of the components of the process as proposed. Experience with using this method or others will provide a sound basis for change, and organizations should constantly reexamine their methods for setting priorities. When making any changes, these groups should consider carefully whether modifying a given element might adversely affect the performance of the entire process.

In proposing a strategy for an optimal priority-setting process, the committee realizes that funding for technology assessment is already constrained and that its proposed priority-setting system will require some additional resources. Given the potential value of priority setting, however, the funding for this effort appears to be justified.

The committee views its report as a strategic effort to look ahead to reasonable goals for AHCPR and OHTA and to create a process that will be credible, sound, and defensible. During the process of compiling data for the quantitative model, OHTA will create a valuable data base and a ranking of priorities; both will be important resources for other organizations as well as for OHTA itself. Indeed, such a program could lead not only to wise use of public and private resources for technology assessment but also to an increase in public support for the entire technology assessment process.

1

Technology Assessment and the Need for Priority Setting

Clinicians, payers, and policymakers turn to technology assessment to help provide better information—to assist decision making in clinical care, to guide coverage decisions, and to set national health policy. Technology assessment can play a valuable role in the entire process of improvement of health and health care. For example, an assessment may show that the data needed for a complete evaluation of a technology are not available. This finding may serve as an impetus to initiate research to supply the missing information. Similarly, an assessment may lead to changes in practice norms when it yields a conclusion that differs from common clinical behavior.

Deciding which of the myriad medical technologies require assessment—and at what point—is a necessity. Even with unlimited funds, it would not be feasible to evaluate all health care technologies; rather, it would be necessary to identify which assessments should have priority. With limited resources, the need to allocate technology assessment funds is essential, but the choices must be defensible. The purpose of this report is to describe such a process—specifically, a priority-setting process for a federal agency— the Office of Health Technology Assessment (OHTA) of the Agency for Health Care Policy and Research (AHCPR). Its broader objective, however, is to propose a process that has wider applications and general utility to other organizations that must set priorities for health technology assessment. This chapter describes how the establishment of AHCPR supports clinical evaluation and how the expanded role of OHTA prompted this Institute of Medicine (IOM) study. It also discusses the committee that was constituted to respond to this request and the methods and terms used by the committee to develop the process proposed in the report.

EVOLUTION OF TECHNOLOGY ASSESSMENT TOWARD OUTCOMES, EFFECTIVENESS, AND APPROPRIATENESS RESEARCH

Health care technology encompasses a wide range of items and services that support clinical practice; it comprises an extensive number of well-established technologies and newly emerging ones. The technologies may include materials from a variety of industries, adaptations of technologies for use in new health settings, replacement of damaged organs and tissue using new or modified procedures and materials, and systems that integrate and monitor information. In what has been called an American "technocopia," such technologies include numerous new and anticipated applications drawn from space and materials technology, the human genome project, and biological research. These may result in genetic engineering applications and new generations of genetic "super drugs." Other technologies may extend preventive and diagnostic techniques to self-care, home, and ambulatory care settings. For example, biosensors and implantable materials for delivering therapies and monitoring the body, as well as the miniaturization of devices, permit treatment to be moved from the hospital to a patient's home or the doctor's office. This flexibility greatly increases the possible range of settings for care and in some cases may decrease the invasiveness of procedures (e.g., new surgical techniques that use small incisions). Other technologies have emerged from work on artificial intelligence systems and from software that assists in monitoring, diagnosis, and therapy—an example is three-dimensional diagnostic imaging. At a multipatient level in the informatics area, health care technologies include microcomputer-integrated clinical management and information systems (Coile, 1990; Misener, 1990).

Ingenious applications such as these seem to hold great promise, and health care technology is often praised for improving medical care. At the same time, it is blamed for fueling the rise in per-capita health care expenditures (Altman and Blendon, 1979; Schwartz, 1987; Ginsberg, 1990). As the costs of health care continue to increase well beyond the rate of inflation in other sectors of the U.S. economy, society has devised methods to control these costs. Yet across-the-board efforts to control the use of procedures and other health care technologies —for example, through administratively imposed caps or cuts in services and programs—have been accompanied by warnings from some health care sectors about the danger these efforts pose to quality and access to care.

Two separate, but related, areas of research—variations research conducted by John Wennberg and others and appropriateness research conducted by Robert Brook and his colleagues—have led policymakers and health services researchers to argue that efforts to control costs should focus on encouraging selective use of technologies; that is, (1) identifying and then encouraging appropriate uses of technologies and (2) discouraging inappropriate uses. Physicians often disagree about the optimal use of diagnostic tests and treatment even for common conditions and well-established therapies (Mushlin, 1991). Wide variations in uses of technologies (see, e.g., Wennberg and Gittelsohn, 1973, 1975, 1982; McPherson et al., 1982; Paul-Shaheen et al., 1987) are thought to be due, at least in part, to such disagreement and uncertainty about their appropriate use (Eddy, 1984; Eddy and Billings, 1988; Ellwood, 1988; Moskowitz et al., 1988; Holohan et al., 1990). A separate body of published evidence on appropriateness has indicated that a significant amount of money is spent in the United States on technologies that are ill suited to the needs of patients and even at times harmful (Moloney and Rogers, 1979; McPhee et al., 1982; Brook and Lohr, 1986; Chassin et al., 1986, 1987; Merrick et al., 1986; Park et al., 1986; Winslow, 1988a,b; Brown et al., 1989).

Medical leaders are convinced that appropriate medical and reimbursement decision making require a better understanding of the value of new or well-established clinical practices, which might be gained from an evaluation of the outcomes of clinical practices in the settings in which they are used (Fuchs and Garber, 1990). Such efforts toward more rigorous evaluation of medical practice are variously called outcomes and effectiveness research, evaluative clinical science, and clinical evaluation (Lohr, 1988; Relman, 1988; Gelijns, 1990; Wennberg, 1990). Effectiveness research has become an important concept in the rapidly evolving field of technology assessment, which in the past has focused on studies of clinical efficacy.[1] The efficacy approach describes results obtained under controlled conditions with carefully chosen patient populations, indications, and settings. Effectiveness research, on the other hand, measures the usefulness of technologies in day-to-day clinical practice. In addition to the more traditional outcomes measured in clinical trials, such as physiological and anatomical change, effectiveness research focuses on other outcomes that are also relevant to patients and clinicians—for example, health status, functioning, and quality of life. Many people believe that effectiveness research will provide physicians with tools for selecting the patients for whom a technology is most likely to provide benefits that are important in day-to-day living.

---

[1] According to Banta and colleagues (1981), efficacy is a measure of the probability of benefit to individuals in a defined population from a medical technology applied for a given medical problem under ideal conditions of use.

The Effectiveness Initiative and Establishment of the Agency for Health Care Policy and Research

Three recent events indicate the attention and interest being directed by the federal government toward effectiveness research as a way to address the nation's growing concerns about quality, effectiveness, and the escalating costs of health care.

First, in 1988, William Roper, then administrator of the Health Care Financing Administration (HCFA), introduced the Effectiveness Initiative within that agency (Roper et al., 1988; Relman, 1988). This initiative sought to identify "what works in the practice of medicine" and to use this information to improve patient care. Roper and his colleagues described an overall approach with three elements: (1) facilitating the use of the large administrative Medicare data sets to monitor trends in the use of services and to analyze geographic variations in the use and outcomes of services, (2) supporting research, and (3) providing this information to clinicians. In support of this initiative, the IOM held a series of workshops to determine which medical conditions should receive highest priority (IOM, 1989a, 1990a,b,d,e).

Second, in 1988, John Wennberg and others prompted the National Center for Health Services Research and Health Care Technology Assessment (NCHSR) to establish the Patient Outcomes Assessment Research Program. Through this program, NCHSR funded a set of multidisciplinary research studies, focused on particular clinical conditions, to assess the outcomes and effectiveness of alternative health care interventions.

Third, by means of an amendment to the Public Health Service Act in the Omnibus Budget Reconciliation Act of 1989 (Public Law 101-239), Congress established within the Public Health Service the Agency for Health Care Policy and Research (AHCPR), which superseded NCHSR. (For further details on the functions of AHCPR, see the appendix to this chapter.) The legislation relocated the Office of Health Technology Assessment, which had previously been part of NCHSR, within the new agency.

The Office of Health Technology Assessment

The Office of Health Technology Assessment, or OHTA, was and remains responsible for performing health technology assessments in response to requests from HCFA. (OHTA also conducts assessments for the Medicaid and CHAMPUS programs, but these are a small fraction of its portfolio.) HCFA uses the assessments for Medicare coverage determinations. OHTA is located in the Public Health Service rather than in HCFA, the agency responsible for Medicare payments, to reduce any appearance of conflict of interest in technology assessment.

ORIGIN OF THE IOM STUDY

In 1989, the authorizing legislation for AHCPR focused and expanded the agency's role in effectiveness research and defined an expanded role for technology assessment as well. In particular, the legislation directed the agency "to promote the development and application of appropriate health care technology assessments—(1) by identifying needs in, and establishing priorities for, the assessment of specific health care technologies..." (Section 904). This charge, and related technology assessment responsibilities, go well beyond the Medicare program and call for the agency to address issues that will benefit the general public.

This legislation was designed to alter significantly the mission of OHTA. Thus, broadening of its role has required OHTA to devise a method to set priorities for the use of its funds. OHTA does not now have such a process for deciding whether to conduct assessments or reassessments other than those initiated by HCFA and, if so, which ones it should undertake.

In addition to its directives regarding AHCPR, the legislation directed the Secretary of Health and Human Services to call on the IOM to recommend priorities for the assessment of specific health care technologies. In asking the IOM to conduct this study, and in keeping with the legislation, the agency proposed that the IOM effort focus specifically on developing a process for setting priorities for technology assessment and reassessment within OHTA.

The agency requested a priority-setting process that would be viewed as objective, broadly based, and defensible against charges of institutional bias. It asked that the process include criteria to permit it to decide whether a technology had reached a threshold for assessment or reassessment and a method to rank-order conditions or technologies requiring assessment. In developing such a process, however, the committee tried to ensure that the process could be useful to other organizations engaged in priority setting. Given the broad scope and purpose of OHTA's new legislative authority, the committee concluded that if the process was properly designed to achieve OHTA's mission, it could be readily adapted by others for their own particular needs.

Previous Pilot Study of Preliminary Model

The current study has its roots in a 1990 IOM monograph, *National Priorities for the Assessment of Clinical Conditions and Medical Technologies: Report of a Pilot Study* (IOM, 1990f), which presented a preliminary model of priority setting for technology assessment. The monograph was the report of work conducted by the Council on Health Care Technology

(CHCT).[2] Congress authorized the establishment of the CHCT in 1984-1985 within the Institute of Medicine to promote development of technology assessment and coordination of the many technology assessment programs in the public and private sectors (IOM, 1988). To carry out its mandate, the council established panels on methods of technology assessment, on information dissemination, and on evaluation.

In response to a request from the director of the National Center for Health Services Research, the council charged its evaluation panel with setting priorities for technology assessment. In its 1990 monograph, the panel described such a process and its outcome, which it titled a pilot study. It focused on both clinical conditions and technologies rather than exclusively on individual technologies, the historical targets of technology assessment. It also used explicit criteria and a Delphi-like process to compile a list of national assessment priorities. (Chapter 2 describes the pilot study in greater detail.) It is referred to in this report as the IOM/CHCT pilot study to distinguish it from the pilot study work that was performed as part of the current project. When Congress created AHCPR, it asked the IOM to extend the council's pilot effort as a way of assisting the new agency in responding to its expanded mandate.

STUDY METHODS

The IOM began its current effort by installing a 13-member committee in January 1991. The committee members collectively had experience that represented the perspectives of practicing clinicians and those in academic medicine and other health professions; national legislative and health care executive policymaking; pharmaceutical and device manufacturing; technology assessment in academic, medical association, research, and third-party organizations; and the areas of health economics, ethics, insurance, managed care, hospitals, and public advocacy.

Between January and September 1991, the committee met three times. Using the previously published IOM/CHCT pilot study as a starting point for discussion, it reviewed the priority-setting methods of a number of organizations and the quantitative models developed by Eddy (1989) and Phelps and Parente (1990). After outlining a process for priority setting, the committee held a 2-day subcommittee meeting in July 1991 to test this process. It heard presentations, made a brief videotape describing aspects of the process it was considering, and sought reactions from individuals who were familiar with technology assessment methods and the needs of

---

[2] The council was disestablished in the same authorizing legislation that created AHCPR.

organizations that undertake technology assessment. Finally, nine individuals, representing expertise comparable to that on the IOM study committee, reviewed the report in accordance with the policies of the National Research Council.

DEFINITIONS

Terms such as *technology* and *technology assessment* are often used without a common understanding of their meaning. To avoid possible misunderstanding, the committee agreed on the following definitions for its discussions.

Medical Technology

Medical technology encompasses a wide range of items and services that support clinical practice, including "drugs, devices, medical and surgical procedures, and the organizational and supportive systems within which such care is provided" (Office of Technology Assessment [OTA], 1978). The term is often defined by example—electronic fetal monitoring, drug therapy, coronary artery bypass surgery, magnetic resonance imaging (MRI), coronary intensive care management. Whether diagnostic or therapeutic, whether intended for the benefit of one patient or many, the term *medical technology* is used to denote all such activity. Diverse organizations, including the IOM in previous reports (IOM, 1985), have accepted this definition, as did this committee.[3]

Technology Assessment

The goal of technology assessment is to provide information on patient care alternatives to patients and clinicians and information on policy alternatives to policy decision makers. It is based on an explicit analytic framework that is specified before the study begins and is comprehensive in scope; that is, it considers higher order impacts such as direct and indirect, short- and long-term, and intended and unintended effects on populations and society.

There are two main categories of technology assessment. *Primary technology assessment* involves collecting data from or about patients and

---

[3] HCFA defines a health care technology as a "discrete and identifiable regimen or modality used to diagnose or treat illness, prevent disease, maintain patient well-being, or facilitate the provision of health care services" (*Federal Register* 54:4305, 1989). This definition is compatible with the OTA definition.

sometimes the collection and analysis of cost dam; it results in the generation of new information through such means as randomized clinical trials and epidemiologic observational studies. *Secondary technology assessment* uses existing data. Its methods include literature synthesis and meta-analysis, cost-effectiveness and cost-benefit analyses, computer modeling, and ethical, legal, and social assessments.

The term *technology assessment* entered medical and health policy parlance in the 1970s, and from the beginning its intent was to consider the social impact of medical technologies (Banta et al., 1981; Perry and Pillar, 1990); OTA (1982) standardized the definition of medical technology assessment as "the field of research that examines the short- and long-term consequences of individual medical technologies." It viewed technology assessment as "a source of information needed by policymakers in formulating regulations and legislation, by industry in developing products, by health professionals in treating and serving patients, and by consumers in making personal health decisions." This formulation grew out of the ongoing efforts of OTA and the National Center for Health Care Technology to promote this field of study as a form of research that would describe and evaluate the effects of a technology on individuals and society. Key areas of attention—safety, efficacy, and cost-effectiveness—and key areas of impact—clinical, social, economic, and ethical—are retained in the term as it is used today. Programs of technology assessment define their goals and objectives in various ways, but in practice they adhere to the OTA definition. In 1985, the Institute of Medicine defined technology assessment, consistent with the OTA definition and very broadly, as "any process of examining and reporting on medical technology used in health care, such as safety, efficacy, feasibility, and indications for use, cost and cost-effectiveness, as well as social, economic and ethical consequences, whether intended or unintended" (IOM, 1985:2).

Consonant with the emergence of the field of effectiveness research, the most recent addition to the terminology of technology assessment comes from Fuchs and Garber (1990), who assert that the field has evolved from an "old" to a "new" form. The old form emphasized biomedical perspectives, that is, the safety and efficacy of an intervention. The new form has a much broader perspective that draws on multiple investigators, multiple data sets, and diverse methodologies to yield an assessment that is based on a range of values and interpretations of the data. As a result, Fuchs and Garber assert that the "new technology assessment is more challenging, more complex, more controversial, and potentially more useful than the old one." Current approaches to technology assessment embrace considerations of health-related quality of life, return to work, functional social and mental status, and patient preferences (McNeil et al., 1978; Fowler et al., 1988; IOM, 1989b), as well as increasingly refined evaluations of costs and benefits (OTA, 1980) and of cost-effectiveness (Leaf, 1989). Indeed, some authors now assert that the aims of and the term *technology assessment* itself have been subsumed in the more encompassing activity of effectiveness research, which goes well beyond measures of safety and efficacy to encompass the assessment of clinical practice (Fuchs and Garber, 1990; Rettig, 1991).

Reassessment

The IOM committee defined the term *reassessment* literally as a subsequent assessment of a health technology conducted by the same institution or organization that conducted the first assessment. Thus, evaluation of a technology by a second organization would not be considered reassessment, although the information from the first assessment would certainly be weighed as part of any new assessment effort.

In their report on health care technology reassessment, Banta and Thacker (1990) note that technology assessment since the 1970s has been focused too narrowly on new technologies. They urge that assessment be an iterative process over the life cycle of a technology as it is developed, disseminated, becomes obsolete, and is dropped from use.

The issue of reassessment of established technologies or of new uses of older technologies has been growing in prominence. Many urge that new technologies not be adopted unless they are known to provide at least some benefit, and that obsolete uses of technologies be eliminated. Yet knowledge of the best uses of a given technology may be scanty, and the diffusion and pattern of its actual use seldom conform to an idealized conception of a linear flow in distinct stages (e.g., developing, newly emergent, diffusing, well established, and obsolete and fallen from use [Banta et al., 1981; see Gelijns, 1990, for extensive discussion]).

Indeed, the diffusion of new technologies while they are still evolving is both a characteristic of medical progress and the bane of efforts to rationalize selective use. Technologies in wide use often require ongoing modification based on clinical experience and studies to determine and refine their most appropriate application. Further, many established technologies tend to be used for wider and wider indications after their initial introduction, even though those new applications have never been formally evaluated. For example, beta-blockers (beta-adrenergic antagonists) were originally marketed for two indications. They are now approved by the Food and Drug Administration for eight conditions but are used in clinical practice for more than 20 (Gelijns and Thier, 1990). Thus, although the committee did not adopt Banta and Thacker's use of the term *reassessment* to include initial assessments of "technologies already in place," it certainly agrees with the need to assess established and possibly obsolete uses of technologies.

REPORT STRUCTURE

The remainder of the report is organized as follows. Chapter 2 briefly reviews several methods of priority setting and draws from these elements the core features of the committee's proposed priority-setting process. Chapter 3 explains the principles that guided the committee's work.

Chapter 4 presents the committee's recommendations for a priority-setting process. It describes the elements of the proposed process and how the committee proposes that these elements be implemented to determine priorities for assessment and reassessment. Because the process entails activities that are beyond the present scope of OHTA, Chapter 5 examines the implications of the committee's process for priority setting within that agency.

Finally, Chapter 6 summarizes the committee's rationale and recommendations, addresses possible problems, and considers how the priority-setting process developed by the committee might be modified by nonpublic entities. In an appendix (Appendix A) the committee describes the pilot study it conducted to assess the priority-setting process it recommended.

SUMMARY

Clinicians, payers, and policymakers are turning to technology assessment to help provide better information for clinical decision making, to guide coverage decisions, and to set national health policy. Yet the efficient use of resources for technology assessment requires a systematic priority-setting process. In the legislation that established AHCPR, the Institute of Medicine was asked to develop a process and criteria for setting priorities for health care technology assessment and reassessment to assist OHTA in its expanded role within that agency. The establishment of AHCPR itself can be seen as recognition of the need to consider systematically the value of health care services in improving health. This kind of consideration uses measures of effectiveness as a means of better understanding the appropriate use of new and established technologies; the expansion of the role of OHTA to develop a comprehensive process to guide this work is consistent with that goal. The process should also be of value to other organizations that, notwithstanding their differing goals, must develop priorities for the use of limited assessment resources.

APPENDIX: THE AGENCY FOR HEALTH CARE POLICY AND RESEARCH

The establishment of AHCPR is a reflection of concerns about the rising costs of health care, the effect on health care quality and costs of knowing little about the value of many health care technologies, and the consequences of using those technologies inappropriately. As stated in the authorizing legislation for the agency (Public Law 101-239, Omnibus Budget Reconciliation Act of 1989, Title IX, Part A, Section 901[b]), its purpose is to "enhance the quality, appropriateness, and effectiveness of health care services."

Center for Medical Effectiveness Research

AHCPR retains many of the functions and personnel of the National Center for Health Services Research (NCHSR) but has a greatly expanded role and much greater visibility than that agency had. For example, the Center for Medical Effectiveness Research within AHCPR has incorporated the medical effectiveness studies of the Patient Outcome Assessment Research Program of NCHSR and is now funding a set of condition-focused grants and contracts called Patient Outcomes Research Teams, or PORTs. These multidisciplinary teams use methods for making inferences from experimental and nonexperimental data to assess all reasonable alternative practices for a specified clinical condition. Thus, one PORT is investigating the care of patients after acute myocardial infarction; other PORTs are studying outpatient care of the diabetic patient and alternatives in the treatment of biliary disease; another team is examining pre-, inter-, and postoperative alternatives in the care of patients with cataracts. In addition to the multiyear, multi-institutional PORT research, AHCPR also funds other, smaller extramural projects as part of its continuing mission of funding health services research.

Office of the Forum for Quality and Effectiveness in Health Care

AHCPR's Office of the Forum for Quality and Effectiveness in Health Care is assigned responsibility for arranging for the development of clinical practice guidelines. Forum guidelines use clinical conditions as a starting point and often incorporate the products of technology assessment. Currently, topics for guideline development are chosen based on a number of criteria such as prevalence, potential benefits and risks, large variations in practice, costliness, and availability of data. Guidelines presently being developed include care of patients with cataracts in otherwise healthy eyes, care of depressed patients, treatment of benign prostatic hypertrophy, and pain management for patients with cancer.

Office of Science and Data Development

The Office of Science and Data Development is responsible for increasing the quality and quantity of data available for health services research

(Department of Health and Human Services [DHHS], 1990). It supports extramural research, demonstrations, and conferences, and is currently investigating the possibility of linking research-related data from different sources. It also formulates science policy for AHCPR and conducts intramural research.

Center for General Health Services Extramural Research and the Division of Technology and Quality Assessment

Two other components of AHCPR deserve mention. The Center for General Health Services Extramural Research promotes research in three areas: cost and financing, primary care, and technology and quality assessment. The Division of Technology and Quality Assessment supports research that includes development and evaluation of methods for conducting health care technology assessments and identification of factors that influence the development, diffusion, and adoption of health care technologies (DHHS, 1990).

Office of Health Technology Assessment

OHTA assesses the effectiveness of medical technologies that are being considered for coverage under Medicare. When a coverage decision cannot be resolved at the regional level or within HCFA, HCFA may refer the question of effectiveness to OHTA. OHTA's plans for conducting an assessment are published in the *Federal Register*.

Historically, the responsibilities of OHTA have entailed what Blumenthal (1983) has called "knowledge processing" rather than "knowledge development"; that is, OHTA does not perform or contract for primary research. Rather, it collects, synthesizes, validates, and disseminates existing knowledge concerning health care technologies. Originally, it was part of the National Center for Health Care Technology (NCHCT). The center itself, however, lacked constituency support and encountered such strong professional (e.g., from the American Medical Association) and manufacturer group (e.g., from the Health Industry Manufacturers Association) opposition to procedure- and device-oriented technology assessment that budget authorization was withheld and all functions of the center, except OHTA, ceased operations after fiscal year 1981 (only 3 years after the center was created). Subsequently, OHTA became a program within the National Center for Health Services Research. In Blumenthal's view, OHTA survived despite the demise of the NCHCT because of its demonstrated ability to save money for Medicare ($100-$200 million per year; Perry and Pillar, 1990). Thus, strong, although recent, historical reasons locate OHTA in AHCPR with its customary responsibilities of responding to requests for assessment from HCFA.

OHTA Technology Assessments

The procedure used by OHTA in its assessments is explained briefly below. Because the agency uses secondary synthesis of published literature for its technology assessments, a given circumstance for beginning work on any topic is that it must be able to retrieve sufficient data to perform an assessment.

Collection of Information. Once OHTA has accepted a request for an assessment and has formulated the assessment question so that it is scientifically and medically answerable, it publishes a notice in the *Federal Register* soliciting comments within 90 days. The agency reviews these comments (which often total a hundred or more) and also solicits opinions from professional organizations and societies, manufacturers, manufacturers' trade associations, consumer organizations, and practitioners and institutions who perform the procedure or use the device. It sends formal letters of inquiry to other PHS agencies, particularly the Food and Drug Administration (FDA), the National Institutes of Health (NIH), and the Alcohol, Drug Abuse, and Mental Health Administration.

OHTA expects the proponents of a new technology to submit data that demonstrate safety and effectiveness. For technologies such as surgical procedures, the proponents must come forward with convincing scientific studies and not simply expert opinion or anecdote.[4]

Analysis of Data. OHTA uses a graded, hierarchical system for examining evidence that is based on study design. The system is comparable to the five grades used by the Canadian Task Force on the Periodic Health Examination (Woolf et al., 1990). Because data from prospective randomized controlled trials are usually not available, OHTA synthesizes the results of other studies, including "quasi-epidemiologic" data or case studies. Recently, OHTA has put greater emphasis on evaluating the quality of studies and on determining whether the technology results in improved health outcomes for patients. For instance, in assessing carotid endarterectomy, the question examined was not whether lesions could be removed from the carotid artery but how the outcomes for patients with removal of lesions compared with outcomes for patients who did not have the procedure.

Assessment and Recommendations. Assessments are subject to peer review within OHTA and are then forwarded to the FDA, NIH, and other

---

[4] For a technology that is currently covered, however, the burden of proof of ineffectiveness would lie with HCFA and OHTA, which makes removal of coverage much more difficult.

appropriate federal agencies. Assessments generally take from 12 to 14 months. OHTA sends HCFA a memorandum that states whether coverage is or is not recommended. Although these memoranda are not subject to the Freedom of Information Act and thus are not available to the public, the literature synthesis and analysis are published and widely disseminated in the series *AHCPR Health Technology Assessment Reports*. At the time of this writing, OHTA had published 10 reports (9 assessments and 1 reassessment) in its 1990 report series. Report topics comprised four procedures (e.g., no. 1, on liver transplantation), two diagnostic technologies (e.g., no. 3, on electroencephalographic [EEG] video monitoring), three treatments (e.g., no. 8, on salivary electrostimulation in Sjögren's syndrome), a revision based on new clinical trial findings (no. 5R, on carotid endarterectomy), and a reassessment (no. 9, on reassessment of external insulin infusion pumps).[5]

---

[5] One report addressed both diagnosis and treatment, hence the apparent discrepancy in the totals.

2
Methods for Priority Setting

Every organization engaged in technology assessment must choose how to use its assessment resources—either through an informal, implicit priority-setting process or by a more formal method that uses specified criteria and available scientific data. The goal of technology assessment varies with the organization conducting it: a medical professional organization assesses technologies to help its members make clinical decisions; information from technology assessment enables a device or pharmaceutical manufacturer to demonstrate the safety and efficacy of its products; technology assessment in the insurance industry supports reimbursement decision making; integrated health care delivery systems (e.g., hospital systems, health maintenance organizations) use the results of assessments to make capital investment decisions and to adopt common clinical management strategies.

This chapter describes how several organizations set priorities for assessments, summarizes models proposed by researchers, and considers how each might contribute to a model process appropriate to the Office of Health Technology Assessment (OHTA). Taken as a group, the examples are not intended to be an exhaustive survey of priority-setting methods but to indicate the range of approaches and features considered by the committee in developing its model and formulating its recommendations. (Criteria reported by eight assessment organizations when deciding which technologies to assess can be found in Appendix B of the IOM report from the Council on Health Care Technology [IOM, 1990f].)

PRIORITY-SETTING PROCESSES USED BY ORGANIZATIONS

Example 1: Health Care Financing Administration

Bureau of Policy Development

Technology assessment is conducted for many reasons, one of the most common being to support reimbursement policy. Coverage determination issues often surface because technologies are expensive, are likely to raise safety concerns, or are likely to be overused. Third-party payers need to determine whether and at what point to cover new technologies. Although the legislative complexity of Medicare necessitates procedures that are more complex than those of private payers, the function of making coverage decisions is a common one. Requests for assessment to OHTA come from the Bureau of Policy Development (BPD) in the Health Care Financing Administration (HCFA). Because these requests have historically been the genesis of OHTA's workload, it is useful to examine the process that produces them.

BPD becomes involved in a small proportion of all questions related to Medicare coverage, focusing on those that are most difficult to resolve and that are of national significance. (Lewin and Associates [1987] and the appendix to this chapter describe the HCFA coverage determination process in greater detail.) Questions that cannot be resolved at the regional level are referred to the central office, but in most instances, Medicare fiscal intermediaries are able to resolve claims coverage questions within existing national policy or by referring questions to HCFA regional offices. With increasing political pressure on HCFA to have uniform contractor coverage, however, requests to HCFA's BPD are becoming more common.

Once a request for coverage has reached BPD, that office decides if a coverage decision is or is not appropriate. If the question is deemed appropriate for a national coverage decision, BPD prepares a background paper for review by the HCFA Physicians Panel.

Health Care Financing Administration Physicians Panel

The physicians panel serves in an advisory role to BPD. Using a set of implicit criteria (e.g., medical and national significance, potential for high cost and rapid diffusion, uncertainty about safety and effectiveness) and considering the background information provided by BPD staff, the panel decides either to recommend that no national coverage decision be made or to refer the technology to OHTA.

Reevaluation or Assessment of Established Technologies

HCFA might also evaluate a service that is already excluded or covered under the Medicare program. Because most covered technologies have never been assessed formally by OHTA, these evaluations are not reassessments as defined by this committee (although they fit the terminology used by Banta and Thacker [1990]). They might be termed "reevaluation" or, more accurately, "new assessments of established technologies."

The purpose of such assessments is to remove obsolete technologies, clarify inappropriate use of otherwise acceptable technologies, and enhance appropriate use of technologies. Publication of clinical studies may prompt such assessments if the findings are inconsistent with current coverage policy or if a service is considered obsolete.

Currently, a HCFA-proposed rule (*Federal Register* 54:4306, 1989) concerning reasonable and necessary services would treat the assessment of established technologies in the same way as the evaluation of new technologies, except that a notice requesting comments would be published in the *Federal Register* announcing HCFA's intent to evaluate. Interested parties could thus also request reconsideration and submit evidence published after the initial coverage decision.

In summary, issues reach BPD, and hence OHTA, by a process that involves requests for coverage to fiscal intermediaries that have been filtered through the regional offices before reaching BPD. BPD decides from time to time (on the basis of stated criteria) that a technology assessment may be needed, but it does not have a priority-setting process for making these decisions (National Advisory Council on Health Care Technology Assessment, 1988).

Example 2: Private Sector—Pharmaceutical Industry

Criteria for Assessment

Pharmaceutical companies[1] exemplify organizations that need to determine how to use resources for biomedical research and development.[2] The

---

[1] This section is based on information provided by committee member Glenna Crooks.

[2] Innovation in medical devices is a strikingly different process. Innovation in some devices involves radical new capabilities, but most often it involves modifying, upgrading, and improving existing devices by a process in which engineering problems are solved or a technology is adapted for a new use or setting. Innovation often originates with clinicians themselves and seldom depends on the results of long-term research in basic science (Roberts, 1988).

top tier of research-intensive pharmaceutical companies, which comprises fewer than 10 companies worldwide, sets assessment priorities for research, development, and testing of compounds on the basis of a demonstration of scientific and market opportunity. Scientific opportunity includes the likelihood of significant clinical benefit. Market opportunity involves several considerations, including those of the Food and Drug Administration (FDA), market-entry hurdles, stockholders' acceptance of long- and short-term research strategies, and returns on investment.

Criteria for Reassessment

Regulatory agencies worldwide require pharmaceutical companies to conduct continuing studies of their products, including, in some countries, postmarketing surveillance. Determining when reassessment is warranted may also require epidemiologic studies on diseases treated by their products to ensure that condition-related adverse events are distinguished from those that are related to administration of the drug. Other factors related to the clinical and market environment may also prompt industry reassessment. These include new (sometimes called off-label) uses of a product. Any of these activities may require primary data collection (e.g., surveying physicians about their uses of a product) or analysis of secondary data.

Pharmaceutical companies sometimes establish external advisory groups to decide when reassessment is warranted. Reviews may either be scheduled or unscheduled and are sometimes prompted by some external event such as new information in the published literature or reports from the field on physician experience with a product.

Internal Process of Priority Setting

An assessment team of senior managers from the company's basic, developmental, and clinical research divisions reviews and evaluates research and development priorities of specific new chemical entities and potential products. Key research data on each potential product are reviewed at monthly meetings at which the team decides whether to proceed, alter, or discontinue that particular program.

Senior management reviews strategic, or long-range, priorities in pharmaceutical development. A development review team reviews the data on compounds it proposes to develop, together with target dates for delivery of each project, and makes a final decision on development. It is reasonable to estimate that such companies use 1 to 2 percent of their research and development budgets for such strategic planning.

Thus, private-sector pharmaceutical manufacturers conduct assessments in response to several circumstances: when there is a regulatory requirement or when a new compound is under development. In the latter case, scientific and market opportunity are assessed repeatedly so that a timely decision can be made regarding further development.

Example 3: Health Care Provider Organizations

Many other private-sector entities, including medical specialty societies, medical group practices, hospitals, and health maintenance organizations conduct technology assessment. Two of the better-known programs are the Clinical Efficacy and Assessment Program (CEAP) of the American College of Physicians (ACP) and the American Medical Association's (AMA) Diagnostic and Therapeutic Technology Assessment (DATTA) program. Other programs include the Blue Cross/Blue Shield Medical Necessity Project and programs sponsored by the American College of Surgeons, the American College of Radiology, and the Council of Medical Specialty Societies.

The CEAP has been active since 1981. The program seeks nomination of technologies for assessment from the 68,000 members of the ACP who are specialists in internal medicine. The college uses a process in which the CEAP committee members evaluate each candidate topic on each of several criteria. The criteria include

- whether good-quality syntheses have been performed recently;
- the clinical impact of the technology;
- estimates of the aggregate costs associated with the technology;
- relevance of the technology to internists;
- the degree of uncertainty among practicing physicians regarding appropriate use of the technology;
- adequacy of the knowledge base for an assessment; and
- the likelihood that an assessment will result in altered practice patterns (Linda White, Director, Scientific Policy Department, ACP, personal communication, October 1991).

CEAP assessments include new and emerging technologies and common diagnostic tests.

The AMA's DATTA program answers questions about the safety, effectiveness, and clinical acceptance of medical technologies. It assesses primarily new diagnostic and therapeutic procedures and technologies and occasionally reassesses experimental technologies if new evidence becomes available (Lewin and Associates, 1987). DATTA receives requests for assessment from individual clinicians, and it also surveys program subscribers and certain interested groups to elicit assessment topics. It then sets priorities implicitly using three criteria: potential impact on substantial patient population, controversy in the medical community, and availability of scientific data (AMA, 1988; William McGivney, former director of the DATTA program, personal communication, 1991).

Example 4: Institute of Medicine/Council on Health Care Technology Pilot Study

The work of the IOM Council on Health Care Technology (IOM/CHCT) pilot study group is another example of priority setting. As described in Chapter 1, in 1989-1990, the National Center for Health Services Research (NCHSR) charged a panel of the CHCT to develop national priorities for technology assessment. That effort resulted in the IOM (1990f) publication *National Priorities for the Assessment of Clinical Conditions and Medical Technologies: Report of a Pilot Study*.

The pilot study focused on developing a method for selecting both conditions and individual technologies of high priority for assessment. The study considered its final list of 20 conditions and technologies (which was not rank ordered) to be illustrative of its process rather than a definitive list of priorities.

Methods used in the study included participation by providers, insurers, and scientists. The broadest level of participation occurred at the point of soliciting topics for consideration, with a deliberate effort by IOM to reach out to an array of stakeholders. Fourteen assessment organizations representing academic institutions, government agencies, health care product manufacturers, health care provider organizations, and third-party payers— submitted candidate topics that each considered to be of very high priority for assessment. The list was augmented by topics suggested by the committee. IOM staff reduced the long list of suggested topics by combining closely related issues under comprehensive headings; as a result, the pilot study listed priority-ranked conditions and technologies formulated at a high level of aggregation (e.g., "coronary artery disease" instead of "acute myocardial infarction" or "coronary arteriogram").

The committee then conducted two rounds of mail balloting and convened to produce the final list (Table 2.1). Each committee member implicitly took into account several primary and secondary criteria to produce a rank-ordered list of each member's highest ranking topics. Primary criteria ("important and readily quantifiable characteristics") included the potential for an assessment to improve individual patient outcomes, to affect a large patient population, to reduce unit or aggregate costs, and to reduce unexplained variations in medical practice. Secondary criteria represented a "spectrum of factors and issues," including the potential to address social and ethical implications, to advance medical knowledge, to affect policy decisions, and to enhance the national capacity for assessment.

In sum, the committee used explicit criteria and a formal process but applied them implicitly to rate individual conditions and technologies.

Table 2.1 List of 20 Assessment Priorities Generated by the IOM/CHCT Priority-Setting Group (in alphabetical order)

Clinical Conditions	Technologies
Breast cancer	Diagnostic imaging technologies
Cataracts	
Chronic obstructive pulmonary disease	Diagnostic laboratory testing
Coronary artery disease	Implantable devices
Gallbladder disease	Intensive care units
Gastrointestinal bleeding	Organ transplantation and replacement
Human immunodeficiency virus infection	
Joint disease and injury	
Low back pain	
Osteoporosis	
Pregnancy	
Prostatism	
Psychiatric disorders	
Substance abuse	

Note: IOM/CHCT = Institute of Medicine Council on Health Care Technology. Using a two-round modified Delphi approach, the priority-setting group chose 20 national assessment priorities from a list of 496 candidate topics. In identifying these priorities, the group considered alternative medical technologies that may be used for each of the priority clinical conditions and the multiple clinical indications for the priority technologies. This list of priorities represented a preliminary set of *general* assessment areas.

Example 5: Food and Drug Administration

FDA establishes priorities for the evaluation of new drug applications and of information submitted about the safety and efficacy of new devices as they are received. It bases its priority setting on (1) the agency's prospective estimate of the level of clinical need for a new chemical entity, (2) the availability of some existing technology to treat that clinical need, and (3) FDA's best judgment (using a three-point scale) about what the new drug or therapy will add to the therapeutic armamentarium.

FDA reviews all new drugs and biologicals at the "front end" for approval under the authority of the Medical Device Amendments of 1976. That legislation (21 U.S.C. 360c) authorizes the agency to regulate all medical devices to ensure that these products are safe and efficacious. The law created a three-tier classification scheme in which only those devices that pose the most significant safety risks must meet premarketing approval standards equivalent to those for new drugs. A list of devices that fall into each category are listed in the *Federal Register*.

QUANTITATIVE MODELS FOR SETTING PRIORITIES

Two sets of researchers have proposed quantitative approaches to priority setting that use explicit criteria and empirical evidence to estimate the relative importance of assessing a set of technologies (Eddy, 1989; Phelps and Parente, 1990). David Eddy developed the Technology Assessment Priority-Setting System (TAPSS) for the Methods Panel of the Council on Health Care Technology of the Institute of Medicine; Charles Phelps and Steven Parente developed a different type of quantitative model for the same body. The purposes of these models are to structure thinking, identify the relative importance of the different elements in setting priorities, and provide a framework to evaluate the effect of different assumptions on priority rankings.

Example 6: Technology Assessment Priority-Setting System

TAPSS is a quantitative model that combines three variables: (1) the population affected, (2) the economic importance of a technology, and (3) the impact of an assessment on the health and economic outcomes for a population. The impact of an assessment is determined by a chain of events that include the likelihood that an assessment will change the use of the technology, the number of patients whose care will be changed, and the effect of such a change on the health of an individual patient (the "marginal effect"). Eddy's formula includes terms for the size of the population that potentially will be affected, the proportion of the affected population in different regions of the country (e.g., differences owing to geography, practice setting, or access), clinical characteristics of candidate technologies, the "Delta" results (the result of an assessment that can potentially cause a change in the use of the technology), "periods" (change in the use of the technology over time), and the effect of the technology on patient outcomes.

Although Eddy's model does not include specific weights to be assigned to different outcomes, he indicates that weights can be employed in a separate, later step in the process (D. Eddy, personal communication, November 1991). He asserts that parameter estimates should be based on empirical sources, if possible, but that when necessary, subjective judgments should be used.

In another instance, Eddy (1989:499) cautions that the model does not provide precise answers but that it is "more accurate and accountable than attempting to perform the entire exercise implicitly and subjectively."

Example 7: The Phelps-Parente Model

In the Phelps-Parente model, calculation of a priority-setting index is based on three components: (1) aggregate spending (cost/unit x number of units); (2) the square of the coefficient of variation (an indication of clinical uncertainty and differences in practice style); and (3) a term that measures how much the incremental value of an intervention falls with increasing rates of intervention (inverse demand elasticity).

The economist's incremental value curve demonstrates how adding populations for a screening technology or more frequent use of a technology such as breast cancer screening increases the rate of use of a procedure until it is less and less likely to confer benefit. (Although this assumption may be valid in general, it may not be valid in any one specific clinical area; for example, mammography may not, in fact, be used by the population that is at greatest risk for breast cancer.)

This priority-setting model assumes, for the sake of simplicity, that the average rate of use is the correct rate, in part because one cannot know in advance of an assessment whether any other rate (higher or lower) is better. The "right" rate can be thought of as that rate at which incremental cost and incremental value are equal. For communities that are not at this "right" point, the dollar value to consumers of the difference in incremental cost and incremental value is called the welfare loss. One must further assume that much of the welfare loss is attributable to lack of information about the appropriate use of the technology and that appropriate use would, at least to some extent, increase as a result of a technology assessment.

Because the model requires a measure of the unexplained variability in use of a particular technology, a technology must be in widespread use in order for it to be included in the Phelps-Parente priority-setting model. The model is thus particularly applicable to setting priorities for reassessment or for primary assessment of medical activities that are well established, but it cannot inform discussions of emerging or new technology.

Phelps and Parente (1990) used hospital discharge data sets, such as those available from insurance claims data and state hospital data bases, to demonstrate the use of the model. The model could also be applied to specific age- and sex-adjusted rates of procedures within a given diagnosis or hospital admission category. It is theoretically applicable in the ambulatory setting, although outpatient data tend to be incomplete.

In sum, by estimating the welfare loss associated with the absence of information on technology, the Phelps-Parente model offers a systematic way to derive rankings for priority assessment and to quantify the expected gains from eliminating unwarranted variation in medical practice patterns.

SETTING PRIORITIES FOR SPENDING ON HEALTH SERVICES

Example 8: Oregon Basic Health Services Act

Example 8 is not an example of priority setting for assessment. Nevertheless, because the Oregon Basic Health Services (OBHS) Act has some features that appear to be analogous to the IOM committee's priority-setting task, it is useful to compare the two. The purpose of the OBHS is to prioritize health spending by the Oregon Medicaid program by developing a "list of health services ranked by priority from the most important to the least important, representing the comparative benefits of each service to the entire population being served" (ORS 414.036,[4a]4). Services are to be provided beginning with the highest ranked and proceeding down the list as far as the Oregon Medicaid budget allows. Thus, the Oregon process makes judgments about the value of services (a form of "technology assessment"); in contrast, the IOM process seeks to determine which assessments should be conducted first. Whether the Oregon exercise is ethical and has merit has engendered a good deal of public discussion (see Brown, 1991; Etzioni, 1991) and is not debated here. What is of interest, however, are the similarities and differences in approach that might help the committee identify possible pitfalls in implementation of its model process.

The difference in purpose between the two methods means that far more detailed information is needed to decide which services are to be provided (as in Oregon) than to decide which assessments should be done. Like the IOM committee in considering assessment priorities, however, those implementing the OBHS believed it possible to establish a fair, open, and explicit way to dicriminate among an array of possible services and to set priorities for state spending based on the greatest benefit to the health of the public served (Callahan, 1991). To that end, implementers of the OBHS have adopted four process elements that the IOM committee also sees as essential.

First, to estimate potential benefit to the public, the OBHS seeks public participation and uses a broadly representative panel called the Health Services Commission. The commission is composed of five licensed physicians (with clinical expertise in the general areas of obstetrics, perinatal medicine, pediatrics, adult medicine, geriatrics, and public health, including osteopathy), a public health nurse, a social worker, and four consumers of health care. Second, implementers of the OBHS sought public consensus on criteria, or values, to guide its process. Third, the process has sought to estimate the marginal benefit of a given technology (the likely difference in outcome that would result with and without the service). Fourth, the OBHS process includes provision for a test of reasonableness to be applied to its rank-ordered list of services (Sipes-Metzler, 1991).

Two additional issues that are also pertinent to the IOM priority-setting process have had to be considered by those implementing the OBHS: whether some issues are "so preeminent that they must trump their way to the top of any priority list" (Callahan, 1991:83) and how the system can respond equitably to interest groups that disagree with a technology's inclusion or exclusion from the list of covered services.

DISCUSSION

Reactive and Implicit Processes

Many of the above examples of priority setting for technology assessment could best be described as reactive, implicit, and internal. They are reactive in that they respond, sometimes *ad seriatim*, to requests for assessment. They are implicit in that decision making about priorities, although guided by stated criteria, is largely the result of global judgments. They are internal because experienced staff of the organization perform the ranking of the candidates for assessment.

For example, OHTA's role in relation to HCFA has been to respond to individual requests for assessment, using secondary literature synthesis to provide information for coverage decisions. With the establishment of AHCPR, however, OHTA has been given expanded responsibilities that reach beyond responses to such requests. OHTA has been asked (1) to set priorities for initial assessments of new or established technologies that might not be important to or a high priority for the Medicare population, and (2) to set priorities for reassessment of technologies that have been previously assessed by OHTA. In addition, HCFA and OHTA need a way to ensure that technology assessment funds for coverage determination purposes are used as productively and as efficiently as possible.

HCFA's priority-setting method is an example of a reactive mechanism that sifts requests and responds to payers, manufacturers, physicians, or other users of a technology by judging when a threshold of "demand" for technology assessment has been crossed. Widespread publicity, for example, about autologous bone marrow transplantation for metastatic breast cancer might induce demand for assessment of this technology; another example of induced demand for technology assessment might be the development of a new device for cataract extraction for which the manufacturer wants Medicare coverage. HCFA and private insurance companies alike use this priority-setting process, which is reactive and, in general, implicit. In their coverage decisions regarding new and emerging technologies, they may weigh potential expenditures most heavily in deciding which technologies to assess. Both public- and private-sector groups, however, have more candidates for assessment than they can accommodate, and all must operate within resource constraints.

Others in the technology assessment field also set priorities reactively. Professional organizations such as the American College of Physicians respond, in part, to the interests of their members. A manufacturer *assessing* the potential market for a device or pharmaceutical product may be primarily concerned with market size and political and market hurdles such as reimbursement and pricing controls, as well as the magnitude of the clinical need—that is, the likelihood that the company's product will have an impact on clinical care. Academic investigators may conduct assessments based on personal interest in a particular topic or on the availability of funds to support the research (Eddy, 1989).

Strengths and Weaknesses of Reactive Mechanisms

There are strengths to be acknowledged in implicit, reactive mechanisms. Their principal advantages are that they provide a timely response to "demand" and that the "hottest" or costliest issues are likely to be addressed first. A further strength is that this kind of priority setting uses the acumen and professional judgments of staff to identify technologies for assessment; as a result, few personnel and other resources are needed.

Some weaknesses of reactive mechanisms can also be identified. First, to the extent that the selection process is closed, it cannot be examined, challenged, or modified by outsiders. Second, the process is unlikely to take into account all perspectives because input depends on access to those who set priorities. Third, although those who engage in technology assessment may find it appropriate to focus on controversial issues, issues that capture passing public attention can overwhelm the process. As a result, the program may never address worthwhile, significant assessments that would add to the practical scientific base of medical practice. Fourth, although implicit estimates about the importance of an issue are necessary and useful in instances when no valid data are available, an implicit method does not make systematic use of data when they are available. Fifth, because the process cannot be examined, it is less likely to be improved upon. Sixth, because of the concerns about costs of new (and frequently expensive) technologies and the political difficulties involved in assessing established technologies, there is a greater tendency to examine new technologies. In contrast to assessments of new technologies, assessments of established technologies encounter strong economic and psychological disincentives to change practice, especially for practitioners and hospitals that are frequent users of the technology. Banta and Thacker (1990) argue persuasively, however, that technologies should be assessed several times during their life cycle.

The IOM/CHCT Process Compared with This IOM Study

The IOM/CHCT pilot study invited a large set of interested groups to nominate candidate technologies and conditions for assessment. In assembling these technologies for further consideration, the pilot study group emphasized the need to assess alternative choices for diagnosing or treating a clinical condition rather than assessing a medical technology taken in isolation from the medical conditions that constitute its clinical content.

The goal of the pilot study was somewhat different from that of this IOM study, however, and its product differs correspondingly. The product of the IOM/CHCT pilot study was a list of priorities that was intended to be valid for the health of the public in 1990; the product of this study is a method for priority setting that can be used anytime in the future. Unlike the IOM/CHCT pilot study, this report does not assemble a list of the top 20 priorities for assessment; rather, it describes an ongoing process for ranking specific candidates for technology assessment such as might be needed by an organization with limited resources for assessment that was faced with choosing among a series of possible choices. The goal of this process is to marshall and use assessment resources to achieve the greatest improvement in the health of the public. To this end, the process must include operational definitions that can be used consistently by those who implement it.

In a variety of ways, which are described in Chapter 4, the method presented in this report is more objective, explicit, and verifiable than that of the IOM/CHCT pilot study. Thus, this study differs from that study but has clearly evolved from it, and this committee acknowledges the path-breaking efforts of the earlier IOM/CHCT panel and the ideas described in its report.

Analytic Models

Both the Eddy and the Phelps-Parente analytic models specify criteria to be used in setting priorities and a formula for combining them; both emphasize the use of empirical data. The Phelps-Parente model uses only available epidemiologic, claims, and practice variation data, whereas TAPSS entails subjective estimates, including estimates of the probability that information will change behavior. Both models start with health care technologies (rather than conditions): the Phelps-Parente model uses established technologies, and TAPSS includes both established and new technologies.

Strengths and Weaknesses of Analytic Models

Analytic models for priority setting share a number of features. The strengths of quantitative models are that they structure thinking, use data (including, eventually, the more humanistic measures of health status that are becoming available), open the process to review and accountability, and are amenable to examination and adjustment not only of the results but of the methodology itself. Overall, they move the technology assessment process closer to a realization of its potential for strengthening the scientific basis for decision making.

The use of models, however, is more complex and requires more resources and expertise than an implicit process that reacts to requests for technology assessment. Furthermore, analytic methods that simply insert values into a formula can be perceived as mechanistic and insensitive to human concerns. Another potential issue is that the use of data and ratings, even though subjectively derived, can appear more precise and authoritative than is warranted. Because the assessment process will affect allocation of resources, the social and political values that will influence recommendations must also be addressed. For both these reasons, the committee emphasizes that any analytic model should use public input and professional judgment about the relative importance of criteria, the science base, clinical issues, and the political environment. It is also important to stress that the priority rankings established by means of an analytic model are inputs to a final decision process, not the final product of the process itself.

Need for a Comprehensive, Proactive Process for Priority Setting

What sort of process, then, would best serve the public interest? Although each assessment organization has its own goals, the public as a whole has an interest in the effects and use of medical technologies. Public agencies need a comprehensive, proactive process of public input to ensure the greatest gain to the health of the public from such technologies.

The priority-setting process must be accountable to the public. It cannot be private, implicit, or internal to the organization conducting the assessment, and it must include a process to identify possible topics for action. OHTA's domain of possible topics for assessment is vast and includes many unevaluated procedures and devices whose original approval was based largely on physician acceptance as determined by decentralized fiscal intermediaries. The agency must have a process not only to respond to requests for assessment but to identify possible candidates on its own—technologies that axe newly emerging, existing technologies whose indications for use need better understanding, and technologies that may be obsolete.

The identification of technologies that should be assessed requires a process that is free of bias. Determining those candidates that should have highest priority seems, like the assessment itself, to require a combination of scientific rigor and consideration of social values. An examination of the principles of priority setting for a public agency is useful in identifying the critical elements of a comprehensive proactive process. Chapter 3 considers these principles.

SUMMARY

This chapter described several examples of priority setting: (1) HCFA; (2) a research-intensive pharmaceutical company; (3) the CEAP program of the American College of Physicians and the DATTA program of the AMA;

(4) the priority-setting process used by the IOM's Council on Health Care Technology in its pilot study; (5) the FDA; two examples of quantitative models of priority setting—(6) David Eddy's Technology Assessment Priority-Setting System and (7) the Phelps and Parente model; and (8) the process developed under the Oregon Basic Health Services Act to set priorities for Medicaid spending.

The committee drew on these examples to derive a set of principles for developing a process for OHTA to use in setting priorities. Although individual assessment organizations may have various goals in assessment, the public as a whole has an interest in the effects and use of medical technologies. Public agencies need a comprehensive, proactive process of public input to ensure that technology assessment provides the greatest gain possible to the health of the public. In addition, priority setting must be accountable to the public. It cannot be private, implicit, or internal to the organization but must include a process that is open, fair, and credible to discriminate among the array of possible technologies it might assess or reassess.

There are a number of benefits to be derived from the use of analytic models—they structure thinking, use what data are available, and open the process to review and accountability and to examination and adjustment of both the results and the methodology. Such models move the technology assessment process closer to a realization of its potential for strengthening the scientific basis for decision making. The use of analytic models, however, is more complex and requires more resources (at least initially) and expertise than an implicit process that simply reacts to requests for technology assessment. The committee also concluded that any analytic model must include a process to review its product and a way to address issues of equity and unusual ethical and legal dimensions presented by health care technologies. Nevertheless, priority rankings established by means of an analytic model should be understood as inputs to a final decision process, not the final product of the process itself.

APPENDIX: MEDICARE COVERAGE DECISION MAKING

The Medicare program, which serves 33 million elderly and disabled beneficiaries and persons with end-stage renal disease, is the responsibility of the Health Care Financing Administration of the Department of Health and Human Services (DHHS). The Medicare statute provides broad authority to cover "reasonable and necessary procedures," but it does not provide an all-inclusive list of specific items, services, treatments, procedures, or technologies covered by Medicare; specifically, it does not list which medical devices, surgical procedures, or diagnostic or therapeutic services should be covered or excluded from coverage (*Federal Register* 54:4304, 1989).

When the Medicare law was enacted, Congress vested in the Secretary of Health and Human Services the authority to make decisions about which services are "reasonable and necessary" to diagnose or treat illness or injury or to improve function. Those statutory terms—translated in practice to "safe and effective," and neither "experimental" nor "investigational," based on authoritative evidence or general acceptance in the medical community—became the basis for payment (coverage) determinations. Over time, of course, many new technologies and procedures have been covered.

"Experimental" and "investigational" technologies are, as noted above, not covered by HCFA (nor, typically, in the private sector); definitions of these terms, however, are variable and murky. There is increasing pressure to pay for (and thus assess) technologies that are not yet standard, established therapies (e.g., investigational Class C drugs for AIDS patients, which are approved by the FDA as investigational new drugs).

Coverage decisions are made in several ways—by local intermediaries and by HCFA with and without an OHTA assessment. HCFA contracts with local, primarily insurance, companies, to process and pay insurance claims from beneficiaries and providers. For Medicare Part A (the Hospital Insurance Program), these payers are known as fiscal intermediaries (FIs); for Part B (the Supplementary Insurance Program), they are referred to as carriers. HCFA issues "national coverage decisions" regarding new technologies and procedures, sometimes after seeking a recommendation from the Public Health Service (PHS) and OHTA.[3] Such decisions then become national policy.[4] Coverage determinations are published in the *Medicare Coverage Issues Manual* and its accompanying instructions. HCFA issues this manual to the FIs and carriers for claims adjudication and payment and to Medicare peer review organizations (PROs) for utilization and quality review. For the most part, however, HCFA gives the FIs, carriers, and PROs broad discretion on coverage determinations, and there is correspondingly variation in what they actually accept and pay for (Lewin and Associates, 1987). Some of the lack of uniformity has been attributed to the absence of a legally binding compliance requirement, to insufficient information about specific technologies, and to difficulty in understanding HCFA

---

[3] A technology is considered generally accepted if (1) research and investigations are complete, (2) the technology has demonstrated value for diagnosis or treatment, (3) it is in general use for patient care, and (4) if relevant, it has been approved by the FDA (although FDA approval is not required for all devices).

[4] The Omnibus Budget Reconciliation Act of 1987 requires quarterly *Federal Register* notices that list all manual instructions, interpretative rules, statements of policy, and guidelines of general applicability to the Medicare and Medicaid programs. Coverage decisions do not normally require notice-and-comment rule making.

coverage instructions. The process has been the subject of recommendations for improvement (Kinney, 1987; Lewin and Associates, 1987; National Advisory Council on Health Care Technology Assessment, 1988).

The Office of Inspector General (OIG; 1990) also found that carriers have difficulty identifying new technologies and are inconsistent in coverage of new technologies that are identified. According to structured interviews and written information, one-third of carriers have experienced major problems identifying new technologies; they depend most frequently on physician inquiries and less frequently on claims submissions. Often, new technologies are not identified because they are given the claims payment codes of current technologies. A new technology may be identified when it does not fit payment instructions, when it is uncoded, when it is given an unrecognizable code, or when the level of reimbursement is challenged by the physician. Manufacturers are sometimes a source of identification.

In the case of FIs, although some consider patient benefit, safety, and effectiveness in making coverage decisions, 73 percent of those interviewed used professional acceptance as a major criterion when making decisions. Fewer than 10 percent of FIs who were interviewed cited cost-effectiveness as a major criterion. The OIG report recommended that HCFA cooperate with the PHS in proactively and routinely compiling information on new health care technologies and rapidly disseminating it.

During any given year, contractors, Medicare beneficiaries, physicians, equipment manufacturers, public officials, professional associations, or government entities request national coverage policy determinations for some 20 to 30 different technologies. The Coverage/Payment Technical Advisory Group (TAG), composed of medical directors and other officers of the carriers and intermediaries, also raises coverage questions.

All such requests go to the Bureau of Policy Development (BPD) in HCFA. Once a question of coverage has been raised, BPD considers a technology for national policy determination if it meets one or more of the following criteria (*Federal Register* 54:4305 and 4318, 1989):

1. The technology represents a significant advance in medical science.
2. It can be described as a new product (for which there is no similar technology already covered by Medicare).
3. The technology is likely to be used in more than one region of the country.
4. It is likely to represent a significant expense to the Medicare program.
5. It has the potential for rapid diffusion and application.
6. There is substantial disagreement among experts regarding the safety, effectiveness, or appropriateness of the technology.
7. The technology has been treated inconsistently by different contractors and fiscal intermediaries, and a conflict can be resolved only by a national decision.

8. The technology was commonly accepted in the past but appears to have become outmoded or its safety and effectiveness are in question.

If BPD decides that a coverage decision is *not* appropriate (for instance, the technology applies to a very rare medical condition or is still in an emerging, preliminary form), that office may still provide information to contractors, which is not binding on their decision, about the opinion of other third-party payers, specialty societies, or recognized medical authorities. If the question *is* deemed appropriate for a national coverage decision, BPD conducts a literature search, consults with the Food and Drug Administration (FDA) on the status of any FDA action, and meets with interested parties. Finally, BPD staff prepare a background paper for review by the HCFA Physicians Panel.

The Physicians Panel (composed for the most part, of HCFA physician employees) serves in an advisory role to BPD—the panel cannot itself make a coverage determination. After considering the background information, the panel decides whether (1) to recommend that no national coverage decision be made, (2) to refer the technology question to OHTA on an "inquiry" basis,[5] or (3) to refer the technology to OHTA for a full assessment.

The following criteria are among those used to decide whether to refer a coverage question to OHTA for assessment (*Federal Register* 54:4306, 1989):

- significant expenditure (e.g., potential for rapid diffusion to a large patient population or high costs on a per-case basis);
- adequate scientific data base; and
- prior FDA approval if relevant (i.e., the technology is a drug, biologic, or medical device that requires approval).

In 1986, the Administrative Conference of the United States recommended that DHHS introduce more "openness and regularity into the procedure for issuing 'national coverage decisions' pertaining to new medical technologies and procedures ... [and] in the process by which the HHS Office of Health Technology Assessment supplies recommendations to HCFA. . ." (*Federal Register* 51:46987-46988, 1986).

In the *Federal Register* of April 29, 1987, HCFA described its process for making coverage determinations and sought comments. In January 1989, following a legal challenge arising from a Medicare coverage issue (*Jameson v. Bowen*, C.A. No. CV-F-83-547-REC USDC [E.D. Cal.]), HCFA issued a

---

[5] The panel might make a recommendation for an OHTA "inquiry" if it is unsure whether sufficient evidence is available or if only limited information is needed.

proposed rule to establish criteria and procedures by which health care technologies could be considered "reasonable and necessary" (*Federal Register* 54:4302-4318, 1989). The proposed rule solicited comments on, among other topics, (1) criteria for coverage decisions and "the identification and selection of health care technologies for national coverage decisions," and (2) "methods for assuring appropriate public participation in the various phases of the technology assessment process."

The rule also proposed that cost-effectiveness of technologies be a criterion for coverage (see Leaf, 1989). At the time of this writing, the proposed rule is still pending. Based on the Notice of Proposed Rule Making, the final rule will likely require not only that a technology be reasonably safe, demonstrably effective, noninvestigational, and acceptable to the medical community, but also cost-effective.

3
Guiding Principles

This chapter describes general principles that underlie the development of any priority-setting process and the implications of those principles for priority setting in the Office of Health Technology Assessment (OHTA).

BUILDING A MODEL PROCESS FOR SETTING PRIORITIES

A process is useful to the extent that it addresses four issues:

- The process should be consistent with the mission of the organization that is to use it. A process that does not incorporate the basic value system of the user cannot help an organization set priorities according to its values.
- The results of the process should be consistent with the needs of the user and should provide information in the form that is most useful. For instance, clinician users of technology assessments seek comparative information based on a given clinical condition to help them in decision making. This issue is discussed further in a later section of this chapter.
- The process should be efficient, especially in instances in which it must share resources with technology assessment itself.
- The process should be capable of operating in the real world of the organization. If the information it produces is to be used effectively, the process must consider not only what information is needed but also the political, economic, and social constraints that will affect how the information can be used.

These principles apply to any priority-setting process. The next section considers how they should guide the development of a priority-setting process for OHTA in particular.

PROCESS BUILDING FOR OHTA

The Process Must Reflect the Mission of OHTA

OHTA's priority-setting process must ensure that the priority rankings it produces are consistent with the agency's objectives. What are those objectives?

The goals and objectives of OHTA are those of a public agency charged with producing information about a medical technology. The information should support the public interest, and OHTA's process should provide the information as efficiently and effectively as possible.

Although specifying the public interest is not an appropriate task for this committee, there is little question that society has expectations of its health care system. An understanding of these expectations is relevant to the work of OHTA and should be incorporated in its proposed model of priority setting. These expectations are related to beliefs about what health care is to achieve and how the health care system is to achieve it—with beneficence, nonmaleficence, and fairness (the goal of distributive justice in the allocation of all resources).[1]

Four elements of the public interest deserve consideration in determining which set of technologies should take precedence when assessment resources are limited:

- the extent to which health care services can reduce pain, suffering, and premature death; increase health, functional capacity, and life expectancy; or maintain the functioning of those who are permanently impaired;

---

[1] In the bioethics lexicon, these requirements are often referred to as duties of the following sorts:
 • *beneficence*, to promote good care (or as it is sometimes expressed, do to others their good);
 • *nonmaleficence*, to prevent or avoid harms;
 • *autonomy*, the general duty to respect persons or, in its applications in health care, the duty to respect the right of self-determination regarding choices about one's life, mind, and body;
 • *justice*, not to discriminate on the basis of irrelevant characteristics (sometimes expressed as treating individuals [or equals] equally in morally relevant situations) or, more specifically and commonly, *distributive justice*, the duty to distribute health care resources in ways that are defensible, fair, not arbitrary, and not capricious (in other words, equitable).
 This discussion is taken from the forthcoming IOM report *Guidelines for Clinical Practice: From Development to Use.*

- the extent to which expenditures for health care services that are ineffective or needlessly costly can be reduced or eliminated;
- the extent to which inequities in access to effective health care services or maldistribution across equally needy populations can be reduced; and
- the extent to which other special social issues can be informed by assessment.

The implications of these elements with respect to a process for priority setting are considered below.

Potential to Reduce Pain, Suffering, and Premature Death

A primary objective of health care is alleviating and preventing the pain and suffering that are part of illness and preventing premature death. Technology assessment—as a primary source of information about the extent to which health care services can effectively achieve these ends—plays a critical role in supporting this primary objective. It should be a priority to the extent that it can lead to the delivery of care that accomplishes these ends.

At a population level, these goals can be viewed as related to the current aggregate burden of illness (the number of people with the condition multiplied by the burden of illness), which is also a measure of the potential for improvement—the medical gain that would follow a change in practice that might follow an assessment. But technology assessment will not necessarily lead to a change in practice solely as a result of providing information on a technology's effectiveness. Such information is only one factor in determining how a technology is used; third-party reimbursement, the practice environment, and legal concerns also influence practice. Because, in the short run, technology assessment affects only the information base of health care decision making, evaluating a technology should not have high priority if increasing information is unlikely to lead to a change in practice. In other words, when any change in practice is unlikely to occur, resources for evaluation should be directed elsewhere.

Potential to Reduce Inappropriate Health Care Expenditures

Although reducing pain, suffering, and premature death is a primary objective of health care, it cannot be considered or accomplished outside of the context of public concern about the magnitude of current health care expenditures and the rate at which they are increasing. This concern suggests that the public would be additionally served to the extent that a technology assessment leads to appropriate reductions in the cost of health care services. Such reductions could follow when an assessment shows that certain health care services are truly ineffective or that competing technologies are potentially substitutable (with no important difference in health gains) at lower costs.

Expenditures for a health care service ought to affect its priority for technology assessment. The important factor for priority setting, however, is not the dollars spent but the potential for more appropriate expenditures. Any reduction in costs depends on the likelihood that cost-saving changes in practice will follow an assessment.

Potential to Reduce Inequity and Inform Other Social Issues

A reasonable goal of any health care system is to deliver the best possible health care to all citizens, regardless of their social, political, or financial condition. This goal is served whenever information is produced that leads to greater equity of health care delivery, especially in terms of the distribution of health care services to those who are underserved, or to more information about a problem that, because it affects a very small population, would not otherwise be the subject of investigation. The priority to be accorded an assessment depends not only on the magnitude of inequity but also on the sensitivity of that inequity to better information. Where there is little capacity to change practice through information, the problem of inequitable distribution of medical services or lack of information about technologies used in the care of a sparsely studied condition will be little affected by technology assessment.

The Product of the Process Should Be Consistent with the Needs of Users

Although the immediate user of the priority-setting process will be OHTA, the ultimate users are those whose decisions will be affected by an assessment. Thus, the committee considered the characteristics that would cause a priority-setting process to produce helpful information for those who use it.

The committee approached this issue by trying first to identify the users of OHTA's technology assessments and to understand how they use the information generated by those assessments. First, clinicians use *comparative information* about a technology; users are almost always interested in comparing the characteristics of one technology with another. Second, users are generally interested in the Characteristics of a technology with respect to some specific *clinical condition*. In some circumstances, users may be interested in assessment to help in deciding about the acquisition of an expensive technology that has the potential for use in a wide variety of conditions (e.g., an imaging technology, a multiphasic blood analyzer). Generally, however, users do not need information, for example, about positron emission tomography (PET) in isolation from the condition or conditions for which it is used. Rather, some users will need to know what information PET can provide for a patient with neurologic disease; others will need to know what information PET can provide that will help a physician evaluate a patient with cardiovascular disease.

The committee recognized that questions concerning coverage for specific technologies drive most of OHTA's current assessments and those of other payers. Nevertheless, the committee believes that OHTA needs to reformulate a question such as, "Should PET scanning be reimbursed by HCFA?" to one that is more useful to clinicians (and ultimately third-party payers)—for example, "What is the optimal management or care for the patient with new-onset angina?" This is the kind of question asked by clinicians, and an assessment will have the greatest impact if it can supply the answers that clinicians seek. If technology assessment efforts are to strive to produce patient-specific recommendations, each candidate for assessment must be specified precisely enough for the assessment to serve a clinician's needs.

Thus, the answer to the above question might eventually be tied to a specific patient population—for example, "PET scanning is the most cost-effective diagnostic test to perform for a 68-year-old male, type-II diabetic patient with new onset of exercise-induced substernal burning." Specification at the level of individual patient characteristics may seem only a distant goal of technology assessment, but the health care system must attempt to achieve it if the assessment and its products are to be useful to the clinician and his or her patients (e.g., McNeil and Abrams, 1986). Such detail was unthinkable 20 years ago; it is now, however, possible to state, for instance, that every patient with a head injury who has temporarily lost consciousness does not need a PET scan, magnetic resonance imaging, a CT (computed tomography) scan, a brain scan, and a lumbar puncture. Instead, a protocol derived from decision analysis can specify the most cost-effective diagnostic test or sequence of tests for a given patient.

Yet great care must be taken, in developing clinical practice guidelines with this level of specificity, to ensure that innovation will continue. There is often a learning curve with new technologies, and because data on such technologies are frequently limited, early assessments may provide incorrect or misleading conclusions. Further, data for good evaluations depend on some diffusion of the technology prior to assessment. Any clinical practice guideline needs to include an explicit statement about the quality of supporting evidence and to make allowance for clinician latitude in the face of poor evidence (Eddy, 1989, 1990a,b,c; IOM, 1990c).

The Process Must Be Efficient

Efficiency requires that the priority-setting process accomplish three objectives. First, it must ensure that important issues are addressed. (If an important issue related to the use of a particular technology is never recognized, then that technology may never come to the attention of the priority-setting process.) Second, the process must ensure that relatively unimportant issues are excluded as quickly and as inexpensively as possible. The first objective implies a process that is open enough to minimize the risk of excluding important issues. On the other hand, openness implies that many candidate topics will turn out to have relatively low priorities. An efficient process will eliminate low-priority issues at an early stage of evaluation before substantial resources have been invested in their evaluation. Thus, the process must include a method to reduce the number of topics if both openness and efficiency are to be achieved.

The third objective is to minimize the cost of data collection. A process for priority setting that requires a large amount of highly detailed information is not reasonable, especially given that a high level of precision in setting priorities is probably not necessary. Given OHTA's access to public data sets and to content experts, a process that uses available data and supplements it with expert opinion will be more cost-effective than a process that requires primary data collection. The eventual implementation of a computer-based patient record might allow much more accurate data gathering than is currently possible at a feasible cost (IOM, 1991a).

The Process Must Be Sensitive to the Environment in Which OHTA Operates

A priority-setting process must be acceptable to those whose decisions are to be influenced by it. In the long run, the acceptability of the priority-setting process will depend largely on the validity of the priority-ranked list of conditions and technologies. The design of the process, however, should include elements that will make the process acceptable and credible. First, it must be understandable; people will mistrust any "black box" process. Second, the logic of the process must be open to inspection, and the logic must be clearly and reasonably articulated. Third, the process must be defensible. Because of the competing demands for technology assessment resources, those who assign priorities must be able to justify the process. Finally, the process must be, and must appear to be, objective and fair. If it appears to be sensitive to the influence of special interests, the product of the process will have no credibility and therefore no power. The process should, therefore, be open to input from a broad array of constituencies. Openness and broad input are the most effective means to ensure objective, fair priority setting.

SUMMARY

The committee formulated several general principles to direct its development of a priority-setting process. The first such principle is that a priority-setting process should be consistent with the mission of the organization that uses it. For a public agency, the values of the public that the agency serves need to be incorporated into the process. For OHTA, such a process would require the assembling of information about the potential to improve health outcomes, to reduce inappropriate expenditures, to redress inequity among those receiving health care, and to inform special social issues.

Second, the priority-setting process must consider the information needs of users. The process designed for OHTA should, in general, focus on technology assessment for *specific clinical conditions* and for *alternative approaches* to those clinical conditions.

Third, the priority-setting process must be efficient so that scarce resources for technology assessment are not needlessly consumed in the process of setting assessment priorities. OHTA should seek broad input at the outset but also have some relatively simple mechanism to reduce a large set of candidate topics to a smaller one. The process should also take advantage of available data, or, where data are lacking, of subjective judgments, rather than require the collection of new data.

Finally, the priority-setting process must be capable of motivating decision makers in a politically complex environment; it must be—and must appear to be—objective, open, and fair; it must also invite input from a variety of interested parties and present the logic of the process clearly and carefully to others. The chapter that follows presents a process that the committee hopes can be understood as logically deriving from consideration of these issues.

4

Recommendations for a Priority-Setting Process

Chapter 3 outlined the general principles of a priority-setting process for conducting technology assessments. Such a process should (1) be consistent with the mission of the organization, (2) provide a product compatible with its needs, (3) be efficient, and (4) be sensitive to the political and social context in which it is used. The process proposed in this chapter incorporates elements that the committee believes are in accord with these principles.

First, the committee's approach uses a broadly representative panel, and the priority-setting criteria reflect several dimensions of social need. It is an explicit process that includes a quantitative model as described in this chapter. The process is intended to be open, understandable, and modifiable as experience with it grows. These characteristics are consistent with the mission of the Office of Health Technology Assessment (OHTA) as a public agency.

Second, the process will produce a list of conditions and technologies ranked in order of their importance for assessment.

Third, the process provides for broad public participation in assembling a list of candidate conditions but then winnows the list to identify important topics, using data when they are available and consensus judgments when data are unavailable. The committee believes that this approach will result in a process that is efficient but that still serves the other principles.

Fourth, the committee's priority-setting process is intended to be sensitive to its political context: it is open to scrutiny, resistant to control by special interests, and includes review by a publicly constituted and accountable advisory body.

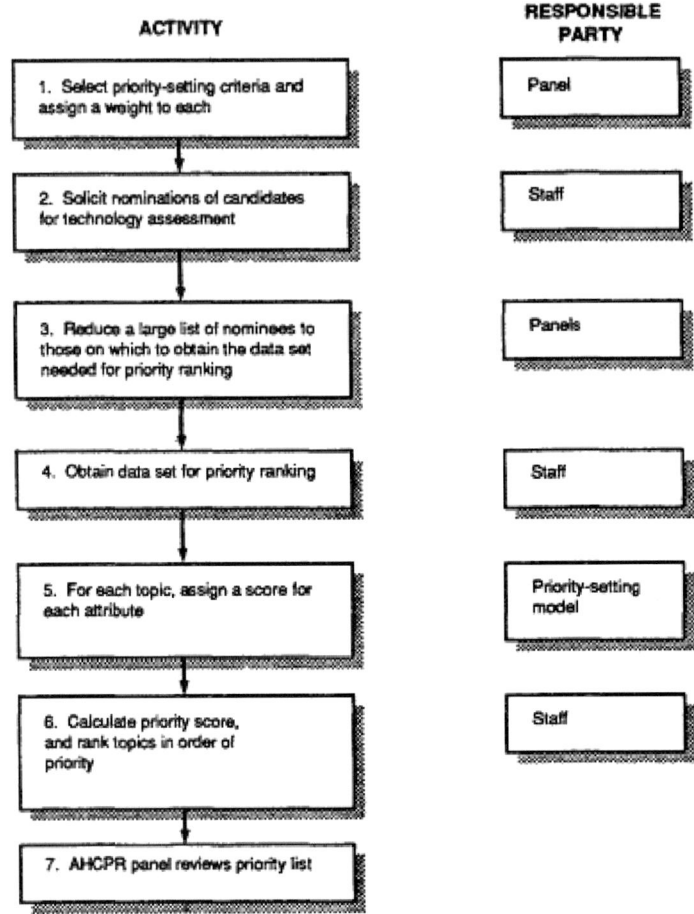

Figure 4.1 Overview of the IOM priority-setting process.

The proposed process includes a quantitative model for calculating a priority score for each candidate topic. In this chapter, the term *process* is used for the entire priority-setting mechanism; the term *model* is used for the quantitative portion of that process that combines criterion scores to produce a priority score.

The model incorporates seven criteria with which to judge a topic's importance. It combines scores and weights for each criterion to produce a priority ranking for each candidate topic. Nevertheless, using the model requires judgments by a panel, data gathering by OHTA program staff, and review by the National Advisory Council of the Agency for Health Care Policy and Research (AHCPR).

During the summer of 1991, the IOM committee pilot-tested its methodology by gathering data on a number of conditions and technologies and using an early version of its model to rank 10 topics. The committee compared two methods of obtaining inputs for the model—a panel meeting and a mail ballot—and modified the model based on this experience. The methods and results of the pilot test are described in Appendix A.

Figure 4.1 is an overview of the proposed steps and participants in the priority-setting process.

PREVIEW OF THE QUANTITATIVE MODEL

The committee's proposed process is a hybrid. It combines features of "objective," model-driven priority-setting methods (such as that of Phelps and Parente [1990]), and a consensus-based Delphi approach, such as that used by the IOM's Council on Health Care Technology (IOM/CHCT) in its pilot study (described in Chapters 1 and 2).[1]

The model combines three components: (1) seven *criteria*; (2) a corresponding set of seven *criterion weights* (W_1 ... W_7) that reflect the importance of each criterion; and (3) a set of seven *criterion scores* (S_1 ... S_7) for each candidate condition or technology. The final "index" of importance of a topic is its priority score, which is the sum of the seven weighted criterion scores (S_i), each multiplied by its criterion weight (w_i).[2]

This priority score or index is calculated as shown in Equation (1) below:

$$\text{Priority Score} = W_1 \ln S_1 + W_2 \ln S_2 + \ldots + W_7 \ln S_7 \qquad (1)$$

---

[1] As noted in Chapter 1, the Council on Health Care Technology no longer exists at the Institute of Medicine. The pilot study described here is referred to as the IOM/CHCT pilot study to distinguish it from the pilot test conducted for the present project.

[2] In the Phelps-Parente model, characteristics such as equality of access, gender-or race-related differences in disease incidence, and similar characteristics have no effect on the overall ranking. Indeed, the output of the Phelps-Parente model was, by design, only one of several inputs into the consensus process that the IOM/CHCT pilot study committee used. In addition, the Phelps-Parente model uses only objective data to measure such things as spending and degree of medical disagreement (as measured by the coefficient of variation). This characteristic is an important limitation to the use of such models, since they cannot be applied when such formal, objective data are unavailable. This drawback may be especially severe when data are limited (e.g., nursing home, home care, ambulatory care) and when new technologies have had little use and have not (yet) been captured in data bases.

where *W* is the criterion weight, *S* is the criterion score, and In is the natural logarithm of the criterion score. The derivation of this formula, an explanation of why the natural logarithm is used, and a description of its component terms are discussed fully in a later section of this chapter.

The model incorporates several forms of knowledge about technologies. The first is "empirical data," such as the prevalence of a condition. The second is "estimated data," which are used when objective data are missing, incomplete, or conflicting (e.g., the number of patients who will use erythropoietin 5 years from now). Third are intrinsically subjective ratings, such as the likelihood that a technology assessment will affect health outcomes.

ELEMENTS OF THE PROPOSED PRIORITY-SETTING PROCESS

The IOM committee recommends a priority-setting process with seven primary components, or "steps." These steps are numbered in Figure 4.1 and are described briefly below; they are discussed in greater detail in the remainder of this chapter. In this discussion, the committee uses the term *technology assessment (TA) program staff* to mean people in a government agency or private-sector organization who are responsible for implementing a technology assessment and reassessment program of sufficient size to warrant a priority-setting process. Similarly, although the term *staff* is used to refer to the staff of OHTA at AHCPR, the term could apply equally to the staff of any agency or technology assessment organization.

Step 1. Selecting and Weighting Criteria Used to Establish Priorities

The first step that OHTA should take is to convene a broadly representative panel to select and define criteria for priority setting. Criteria can be both objective and subjective. The panel should also assign to each criterion a weight that reflects its relative importance.

The IOM committee proposes and later defines seven criteria: three objective criteria—prevalence, cost, and variation in rates of use; and four subjective criteria—burden of illness, potential of the results of the assessment to change clinical outcomes, potential of the results of the assessment to change costs, and potential of the results of the assessment to inform ethical, legal, and social (ELS) issues. Table 4.1 defines these criteria. The justification for each and "instructions for use" appear later in this chapter under Step 5.

Different organizations might, through their own procedures, choose different criteria and assign different weights to each. The IOM committee believes there are good reasons why the seven criteria that it chose are the best for OHTA to select. These criteria and the weights assigned to them are used in a quantitative model for calculating priority scores for each candidate for assessment.

Table 4.1 Criteria Recommended for the IOM Priority-Setting Process

No.	Criterion (Type[a])	Definition
1	Prevalence (O)	The number of persons with the condition per 1,000 persons in the general U.S population
2	Burden of illness (S)	The difference in quality-adjusted life expectancy (QALE) between a patient who has the condition and receives conventional treatment and the QALE of a person of the same age who does not have the condition
3	Cost (O)	The total direct and induced cost of conventional management per person with the clinical condition
4	Variation in rates of use (O)	The coefficient of variation (standard deviation divided by the mean)
5	Potential of the results of an assessment to change health outcomes (S)	The expected effect of the results of the assessment on the outcome of illness for patients with the illness
6	Potential of the results of an assessment to change costs (S)	The expected effect of the results of the assessment on the cost of illness for patients with the illness
7	Potential of the results of an assessment to inform ethical, legal, or social issues (S)	The probability that an assessment comparing two or more technologies will help to inform important ethical, legal, or social issues

[a] O = Objective criterion; S = subjective criterion.

Step 2. Identifying Candidate Conditions And Technologies

To generate the broadest possible list of candidate technologies for assessment, TA program staff should seek nominations from a wide range of groups concerned with the health of the public. These groups include patients, payers, providers, ethicists, health care administrators, insurers, manufacturers, legislators, and the organizations that represent or advocate for them. TA program staff should also track candidate technologies and gather information on relevant political, economic, or legal events; these might include the emergence of a new technology or new information regarding practice patterns for an established technology, a legal precedent-setting case, an assessment of a technology performed by another organization, completion of a pertinent randomized clinical trial, or the appearance of other new scientific information.

Step 3. Winnowing the List of Candidate Conditions and Technologies

Once TA program staff have identified what is likely to be a very large set of candidate conditions, they should set in motion some method to identify the most important topics, using a method to "winnow" this initial list to one that is more manageable. The reason for reducing the list of candidate topics is to reduce the workload of TA program staff (who must obtain a data set about each topic that will be ranked) and to reduce the workload of the panels. Ideally, this process of winnowing will be much less costly than the full ranking system and will be, like the overall priority-setting process, free of bias, resistant to control by special interests, open to scrutiny, and clearly understandable to all participants. The committee discusses several possible methods later in this chapter and proposes one for OHTA and other groups.

Step 4. Data Gathering

When the starting point for the priority-setting process is a clinical condition, TA program staff should define all alternative technologies for managing that condition. In this context, "managing" includes primary screening and prevention, diagnosis, treatment, rehabilitation, palliation, and other similar elements of care. For each condition under consideration, OHTA staff must gather the data required for each priority-setting criterion. Analogously, when the starting point is a technology, TA program staff need to specify the most important clinical conditions for which it is relevant and any other relevant technologies and amass the data required for each priority-setting criterion. The data include numbers (e.g., prevalence, cost) and facts with which to inform a subjective judgment (e.g., a list of current ethical, legal, and social issues).

Step 5. Creating Criterion Scores

At this point, the IOM process calls for panels to develop criterion scores (the S_1-S_7 elements in Equation [1]). One or more *expert panels*, which might be subpanels of the broadly representative panel that sets criterion weights, would determine criterion scores for objective criteria, using the data that have been assembled by TA program staff for each condition. Assigning scores for objective criteria will require expertise in epidemiology, clinical medicine, health economics, and statistics when data are missing, incomplete, or conflicting. One or more *representative panels*, which might be the same individuals as those setting criterion weights, would use consensus methods to assign scores for subjective criteria.

Step 6. Computing Priority Scores

From all these inputs, TA program staff would use the quantitative model embodied in Equation (1) to calculate a priority score for each condition. This calculation is performed as follows: (a) find the natural logarithm of each criterion score; (b) multiply that figure (i.e., the natural logarithm) by the criterion weight to obtain a weighted criterion score; and (c) sum these weighted scores to obtain a priority score for each condition or technology. The quantitative model combines empirical rates (e.g., number of people affected per 1,000 in the U.S. population) and subjective ratings (e.g., burden of illness) for each criterion (each given a certain "importance" by virtue of its particular weight) to produce a priority score. Table 4.2 illustrates the process.

In the second part of this step, TA program staff list the candidate technologies and conditions in the order of their priority scores. According to the model, higher scores will be associated with conditions and technologies of higher priority. TA program staff should also at this time determine whether another organization is already assessing a topic and delete such

Table 4.2 Nomenclature for Priority Setting

Example:
Priority Score $= W_2 \ln S_2 + ... + W_7 \ln S_7$
where W_1 = subjectively derived weight for criterion 1, S_1 = criterion score for criterion 1, and ln = the natural logarithm of the criterion score.

Criterion Name (Type)[a]	Criterion Weight (W)	Criterion Score (S)
Prevalence (O)	W_1	Number/1,000 persons
Cost (O)	W_2	Cost/person
Variations in rates (O)	W_3	Coefficient of variation for rate of use
Burden of illness (S)	W_4	1-5 rating
Potential for the result of an assessment to change health outcomes (S)	W_5	1-5 rating
Potential for the results of an assessment to change costs (S)	W_6	1-5 rating
Potential for the results of an assessment to inform ELS[b] (S)	W_7	1-5 rating

[a] Criterion types: O = objective; S = subjective.
[b] ELS = Ethical, legal, and social issues.

topics from the priority-ranked list for assessment. In addition, staff must decide whether the published literature is sufficient to support an assessment; if it is not, it has a number of options, as described in Chapter 5.

Step 7. Review By Ahcpr National Advisory Council

The seventh and final step involves an authoritative review of the priority list as it exists at the end of Step 6; in the case of OHTA, the AHCPR National Advisory Council would conduct this review. Other agencies or organizations would use other definitive review entities. For simplicity, this discussion focuses on OHTA and AHCPR.

To complete the priority-setting process, TA program staff would provide the advisory council with definitions of the criteria, a list of the criterion weights, the criterion scores for each candidate topic, and the priority list itself. After review and discussion of this material, the council might take one of several actions: recommend adopting the priority list as a whole; recommend adopting it in part and adjusting the priority rankings in various ways; or reject it outright and request a complete revision for re-review. Depending on its conclusions at this stage, the council would then advise the AHCPR administrator about implementing assessments of the highest ranking topics.

DETAILS OF THE PROPOSED PRIORITY-SETTING PROCESS

Step 1. Selecting And Weighting The Criteria Used To Establish Priority Scores

Selecting Criteria

As will be clear from the technical discussions that follow, the criteria established for this priority-setting process have great importance because so much rests on their clear, unambiguous definition and on the weights that are assigned to them. To ensure that this crucial part of the process is given due attention, the IOM committee recommends that a special panel be convened to participate in a consensus process.

This panel would choose the criteria that will determine the priority scores and assign a weight to each criterion. It should broadly reflect the entire health care constituency in the United States because its purpose is to characterize the preferences of society. (The assumption is that, for OHTA, the agency itself would convene this panel. Other organizations might empanel such bodies independently, use the product of an AHCPR panel, or turn to some neutral institution, such as the IOM, to carry out this critical first step.)

The panel would perform this function only once. (Although the IOM committee envisions a face-to-face group process, the criteria might be selected and weighted by means of a mail balloting procedure that uses a formal group judgment method such as a Delphi process. A mailed ballot would require that the staff prepare especially thorough background educational training materials.)

The IOM committee considered many possible criteria and recommends the seven that appear in Table 4.1 and that are described fully in Step 5. Chapter 3 argued that the public interest would be well served by a process that assigned priority based on the potential of the assessment to (a) reduce pain, suffering, and preventable deaths; (b) lead to more appropriate health care expenditures; (c) decrease social inequity; and (d) inform other pressing social concerns. The criteria proposed by the committee address these interests.

Weighting Criteria

Various approaches can be used to assign criterion weights. After some discussion of alternatives, the committee chose the following procedure, which is relatively straightforward and can be easily explained, defended, and applied. The discussion below addresses how to assign weights and what scale to use. It includes a description of a workable group method.

The panel, by a formal vote, would choose one criterion to be weighted lowest, and it would give that criterion a weight of 1. (Any criterion given this weight is neutral in its effect on the eventual priority score.) Panel members would then assign weights to the remaining criteria relative to this least important criterion. For example, assume that criterion A is considered the least significant and is accorded the weight of 1. If criterion C were considered three times as important as criterion A, it would be given a weight of 3.

The scale of the weights is arbitrary. The committee chose to bound the upper end of the scale at 5. Therefore, individual weights need not reach, but should not exceed, 5. Weights need not be integers; for example, 2.5 is an acceptable weight. In addition, the same weight can be used more than once. If a panel member believes that no criterion is more important than any other, he or she would assign to each a weight of 1.

After each panel member assigns weights, the panel would discuss the weights and, depending on the degree of initial consensus, take one or more revotes. The mean of the weights of individual panel members[3] following

---

[3] Because the criterion weighting scale is a rational scale in which, for instance, a weight of 2 indicates twice the importance of a weight of 1, one might wish to use the geometric rather than arithmetic mean. There is, however, no logical necessity for using the geometric mean, and the process of determining social preferences (relative importance) can be carried out in any way the panel finds comfortable. The goal is to have the panel replicate something akin to a "social utility function" showing the importance of various component parts of the priority-scoring model. How those weights are determined does not depend on the mathematical way in which they are eventually used—which, in the committee's model, is in a multiplicative fashion, as expressed in Equation (1).

the second (or last) revote is the criterion weight to be used in Equation (1) for the remainder of the priority-setting process.

Step 2. Identifying Candidate Conditions And Technologies

The second step in the IOM committee's process is to identify a list of candidate conditions. An ongoing function of a technology assessment program is to assemble lists of candidate conditions and technologies. This process includes soliciting nominations directly for a large pool of candidate conditions and technologies, accepting suggestions from usual sources and "customers" of technology assessment, and tracking external events that may affect either the pool or the eventual priority-ranked list.

As a first stage, TA program staff would routinely solicit from a very broad group a list of topics (technologies and clinical conditions) that might be considered for assessment. The IOM/CHCT pilot study assembled a long list of candidate topics using such a process; that list might serve as a source of topics and a taxonomy of technologies for AHCPR and other organizations that conduct assessments.

Simultaneously, the TA program would compile and catalog requests that arrive in the usual manner from the Health Care Financing Administration (HCFA), from the Medicaid and CHAMPUS programs, from practitioners and providers and their professional associations, and from other sources.

Finally, TA program staff would be alert to events that affect the characteristics of a technology, clinical condition, or current practice, including the potential to modify patient outcomes. Events that would put a technology or condition on a list of candidates for assessment are

- a recent rapid and unexplained change in utilization of a technology;
- an issue of compelling public interest;
- an issue that is likely to affect health policy decisions;
- a topic that has created considerable controversy;
- new scientific information about a new application of an existing technology or the development of a new technology for a particular condition or practice; and
- a "forcing event," such as a major legal challenge, or any other event that might raise any of a topic's criterion scores.

Step 3. Winnowing The List Of Candidate Conditions And Technologies

Any process of obtaining nominations that allows for the input of a broad range of groups should lead to a large number of candidate conditions and technologies. When the IOM/CHCT pilot study used this sort of approach, it received 496 different nominations. Because each technology or condition that

RECOMMENDATIONS FOR A PRIORITY-SETTING PROCESS 67

receives a final ranking will require data gathering by OHTA staff and work by the priority-setting panels, it is desirable to find an efficient, low-cost method to reduce the initial list of nominees to a more manageable number. Thus, winnowing the list is the third element of the IOM priority-setting process.

The winnowing step should have several features. First, it should be less costly than the full ranking system; otherwise, it contributes little to the priority-setting process. Second, it should be free of bias and resistant to control by special interests. (For example, no one organization or person should be able to "blackball" a nomination, nor should they be able to force a nomination onto the list.) The process should be clearly understandable to all participants. Possible approaches fall into three groups: intensity ranking, criterion-based preliminary ranking, and panel-based preliminary ranking.

- *Intensity ranking.* The original nominator (a person or organization) would be asked to express some degree of intensity of preference for having individual technologies evaluated. TA program staff would aggregate those rankings and eliminate topics at the lower end of the list before proceeding to a complete ranking of the remaining list.
- *Criterion-based preliminary ranking.* TA program staff would rank all nominated technologies and conditions according to a subset of criteria. They would eliminate some topics on that basis and then proceed to rank the remaining set fully.
- *Panel-based preliminary ranking.* TA program staff would use panels to provide subjective rankings on all or a subset of candidate technologies. Only the highest ranking topics would remain for the full ranking process.

After discussing all three approaches and variants of each, the IOM committee recommends using the last method—panel-based preliminary ranking. A full description of each approach and the rationale for favoring the panel-based method for OHTA are given in Appendix 4.1 at the end of this chapter.

The panel-based method uses one or several panels to provide preliminary (subjective) rankings of the nominated technologies. To minimize costs, these activities could be conducted using mail ballots or (a more modern variant) electronic mail.

Two versions of this process can be described: a double-Delphi system and a single-panel, in-and-out system. The committee does not view one or the other as preferable.

- *Double-Delphi system.* This method would use two panels that might be constituted with quite different memberships. Each would select (for example) their top 150 unranked technologies. The list for priority setting would include only those technologies that appeared on both lists. In an alternative method, each panel would "keep" (for example) 50 technologies,

and the list for priority setting would include those technologies that appeared on either list.
- *Single-panel, in-and-out system.* This approach would use only a single panel that would generate two sets of technology lists. Those topics on the first list (e.g., the top 5 percent of the submitted nominations) would automatically go forward to the next step in the process. The bottom 50 percent of nominations would be excluded from further consideration. The remaining 45 percent (in this example) would go to a second-tier winnowing process that would consist of several more cycles of this process or an entirely different approach, such as a data-driven system.

Secondary Winnowing Processes

Apart from whatever initial winnowing system is used, two other features can enhance any winnowing process. These include provisions for "arguing-in and arguing-out" and requesting or requiring supporting data.

- *Arguing-in and arguing-out.* This tactic allows for an appeal or "re-hearing" to convince others in the process to include or exclude a candidate technology from the final list that will receive complete ranking.
- *Supporting data.* To use this feature, TA program staff request (or require) organizations that nominate candidate technologies and conditions to submit data with their nominations or, at a minimum, references to relevant data; the objective is to obtain sufficient information to allow complete ranking of the technology. For example, submissions might include information on the prevalence of the condition, current costs of treatment, variability of use of the intervention in question, and so forth.

Either of these approaches could be used in combination with the chosen method of winnowing.

Step 4. Data Gathering

The fourth element of the IOM process is gathering data that the panels will use to assign criterion scores. This task first requires specifying the principal clinical conditions for each technology or the alternative technologies used for each clinical condition. The second step is to assemble the required data for each condition and each criterion.

Specifying Alternative Technologies And Clinical Conditions

After winnowing the initial list of candidate topics, TA program staff would specify all relevant alternative approaches for care of a given clinical condition. For example, if the clinical problem was "predicting the course of illness for men with chronic stable angina," the alternative technologies might include exercise stress electrocardiogram, stress thallium scintigraphy, echocardiography, and coronary angiography. For this task, OHTA staff should define clinical conditions to include the most important subgroups (as defined by age, gender, or clinical criteria). Framing the topic in this way must be done with care to prevent the clinical condition from being defined improperly, which might result in its undeservedly receiving a low priority score or its mistakenly receiving a high score.

Staff Summaries Of Clinical Conditions

As a first step in assigning priority scores, OHTA staff would conduct a literature search for each candidate condition and technology to summarize for the panels the data they will need to assign a score to each priority-setting criterion. The panels would use the summaries to make subjective judgments; they would use the objective data (e.g., prevalence, costs, variation in practice) to assign scores to the priority-setting criteria.

Step 5. Creating Criterion Scores

General Points

Criterion scores (S_n in Equation 1) are of two kinds: objective and subjective. Where objectively measurable data (e.g., costs, prevalence) are available, the committee recommends using them. When no objective measure is available or a probability has to be estimated, a panel can create subjective scores in the form of ratings. These distinctions are briefly elaborated here; detailed discussion of the seven recommended criteria follow.

- *Objective Criteria.* TA program staff would collect data for each of the conditions appearing on the list of candidate conditions or technologies. The units in which objective criteria are expressed must be consistent from condition to condition. For example, when counting the number of people affected, one must count "people with the illness," not "people treated for the illness," for all conditions. Similarly, when estimating per-capita spending, the measure must be dollars in every case, not dollars for some diseases and Relative Value Scale units in others. TA program staff should express prevalence as number of persons per 1,000 in the total U.S. population, even for those illnesses that affect only one segment of the population, such as women, a particular ethnic group, or children.

Good information will be available for some disease conditions (e.g., prevalence of lung cancer) but not for others (e.g., prevalence of hemochrom atosis-related impotence). When objective data are not available or are conflicting, or when a criterion requires combining several measures with different units, the panel can use a formal group process to estimate missing information and resolve conflicting data; the IOM committee's pilot-test subcommittee did just that (see Appendix A).

Members of the panel engaged to assist with the objective criteria might be a subpanel of the criteria weighting panel. The subpanel would include epidemiologists, statisticians, health economists, and health care practitioners.

- *Subjective Criteria.* The committee proposes using subjective estimates or ratings when no objective measure is available or when probabilities must be estimated. An example of a subjective criterion is the likelihood that health outcomes will change as a result of an assessment. A formal consensus process provides a good way to perform this estimation.

The panel engaged to assign subjective criterion scales would be constituted differently from the panels for creating the "objective criterion scores." The panel should be broadly representative and include a range of health professions as well as users of health care.

Each subjective criterion score can be represented by a rating on a scale of 1 to 5 (the length of the scale is arbitrary). If possible, the ends of the scale should be defined for each criterion. The panel for assigning scores for subjective criteria would use these scales to create "criterion scores" (ratings), which are inputs into the priority score calculation in the same way that objective data are inputs.

The magnitude of a topic's criterion score reflects the topic's priority for technology assessment. Scores between 1 and 5 will increase a topic's priority for assessment. A score of 1 has no effect on priority, no matter what weight is chosen, because the natural logarithm of 1 is zero, and the contribution of the criterion to the priority score is obtained by multiplying the criterion weight by the criterion score.[4] (Recall that the priority score is calculated as: $PS = W_1 \ln S_1 + W_2 \ln S_2 + ... + W_7 \ln S_7$.)

There are two methodologic issues to be resolved in setting the upper and lower bounds for the subjective criterion scores: first, whether to set the bounds in a one-stage or a two-stage process, and second, whether

---

[4] The committee considered a symmetrical scale that would run from (for instance) 0.2 to 5 to allow the subjective criterion scores to lower the priority of a technology for assessment. Scores of less than 1 but greater than 0 would reduce a topic's priority score because the natural logarithm of a number less than 1 is a negative number. In a multiplicative scoring system, a criterion score of 0.5 (1/2) would reduce a priority score by the same proportion that a score of 2 increases a priority score (e.g., the natural logarithm of 2 is 0.693, and the natural logarithm of 0.5 is -0.693). Similarly, scores of 0.333 (1/3) and 3 would have corresponding effects, as would scores of 0.25 (1/4) and 4, and 0.2 (1/5) and 5. However, because the objective criteria, costs and prevalence, unlike the subjective criteria, cannot be negative, the committee decided to use a single positive scale that runs from 1 to 5 for all subjective criteria.

scores must be comparable from one priority-setting cycle to the next or from one organization to the next.

First, for a one-stage process, each panel member might independently choose a highest ranking condition or technology and assign it a rating of 5; similarly, each member could do the same for the lowest ranking technology or condition and assign it a 1. Each panel member would then set the scores for the other criteria. The committee believed, however that this task should be done in a two-stage process. After the panel decides on the highest and lowest rated conditions or technologies, each panel member would then individually assign scores to the remaining topics.

Second, there are several alternative ways to define the ends of the scale for a subjective criterion. It is possible to anchor the ends of the scales independently of a particular set of topics to be assessed and a particular technology assessment organization. There are advantages to this system in allowing consistency over time and from one organization to the next. The committee believed, however, that the need to spread ratings across the entire scale outweighed the possible virtues of comparing across organizations; thus, it recommended anchoring the scales with the high- and low-rated condition each time priorities are established.

Criteria Recommended For The Iom Priority-Setting Model

The committee recommends seven criteria for use in its model (see Table 4.1). The first three criteria form a set that estimates the aggregate social burden posed by a candidate clinical condition. The first criterion considers the general population afflicted with the condition, that is, its *prevalence*. The second and third criteria consider the burden to the patient, or the *burden of illness*, and the economic burden, or *costs*.

The fourth criterion, *variation in rates of use*, addresses clinical practice and the possible role of uncertainty on the part of health care providers about the best way to manage the clinical problem.

The Fifth, sixth, and seventh criteria also form a set. They consider the possible effect of the results of the technology assessment itself: whether the results of the assessment are likely to *affect health outcomes, affect costs*, or *inform ethical, legal, and social concerns*. These seven criteria are described in greater detail below.

Criterion 1: Prevalence

Definition: Prevalence is the number of persons with the clinical condition per 1,000 persons in the U.S. general population. This definition applies to assessments of a clinical condition and to assessments of a technology.

Comments. As applied to assessing a technology, this definition presupposes an assessment of the technology's application to relevant clinical conditions. If the technology is applied to more than one condition, prevalence should be the sum of the prevalence of the individual conditions, each weighted by the relative frequency with which the technology is used for that condition.

To maintain consistent units for this criterion, which is one of the objective criteria in this process, the time frame for measuring them must be the same. There are two alternative but equivalent ways to define prevalence and the other objective measure of social burden, the cost of care. In one, the time horizon is one year. Thus, prevalence is the number of cases per 1,000 persons in the U.S. general population, and costs are annual expenditures. In the other, the time horizon is the length of the illness. "Prevalence,"

Table 4.3 Consistent Units for Prevalence Criterion, by One Year and Lifetime Time Horizons

Criterion	Two Time Horizons	
	One Year	Lifetime
Prevalence	Prevalence	Incidence
Cost	Annual	Lifetime[a]
Variations in rates of use	Coefficient of variation	Coefficient of variation
Burden of illness	Change in quality-adjusted life days in the next year as a result of illness	Change in quality-adjusted life expectancy due to illness[a]
Potential of the results of an assessment to change health outcomes	Expected change in outcomes in the next year as a result of assessment	Expected change in outcomes over average patient's lifetime owing to assessment[a]
Potential of the results of an assessment to change costs	Expected change in costs in the next year as a result of assessment	Expected change in costs over average patient's lifetime as a result of assessment[a]
Potential of an assessment to inform ethical, legal, and social issues	Expected change in ELS[b] issues in the next year	Expected change in ELS issues in the next year

[a] Requires a consistent discount rate.
[b] ELS = Ethical, legal, and social issues.

then, is the number of people who acquire the illness per year (in other words, the incidence of the condition), and costs are the lifetime costs of the condition. Table 4.3 indicates units for the prevalence criterion that are consistent for the two possible time horizons, per year (which uses actual prevalence) or lifetime (which uses incidence).

Using either approach requires the analyst to determine the relevant denominator for estimating prevalence and to use that same measure as the denominator for all candidate topics. If a particular age range, gender, or other characteristic of the population at risk is not specified, all conditions and technologies assume an equivalent basis for determining national priorities. Organizations thus should not define the denominator in terms of a particular population at risk, lest the condition receive too much weight relative to a condition whose prevalence is expressed in terms of the general population.

Determining the numerator for procedures and tests is another important methodologic issue. Whether the rate of testing is defined as the current rate or the projected rate may depend on the particular condition for which the technology is relevant. If the incidence of disease is changing rapidly, using projected rates may be appropriate. When evaluating a technology for which indications are changing, identifying the correct at-risk population is important. For instance, if erythropoietin were a candidate technology, assessors would need to determine whether the population of interest is all patients with anemia, those with anemias of chronic illness, or those with anemia due to renal failure. Prevalence must be expressed in terms of the general population to be consistent with the denominator and to maintain consistency among candidate topics.

Data Sources. These data can be found in Medicare or insurance company data files or in survey data compiled by the National Center for Health Statistics.

Criterion 2: Burden Of Illness

Definition. Burden of illness is the difference in quality-adjusted life expectancy (QALE) between a patient who has the condition and who receives conventional treatment and the QALE of a person of the same age who does not have the condition.

Comments. This definition applies to assessments of a clinical condition and to assessments of a technology. Although some data on mortality and morbidity are available, at present these data are seldom obtainable at the level of specificity needed; consequently, the panels will have to assign criterion scores by a subjective estimate of the burden of illness of one candidate clinical condition as compared with the others. QALE is the product of life expectancy and quality of life. Examples are given in Figures 4.2 and 4.3.

The best measure of burden of illness is the change in quality-adjusted life expectancy attributable to a condition, because this unit of measure takes into account both mortality (shortened life expectancy) and morbidity (quality-of-life adjustment factors). As applied to assessments of a technology, the definition of burden of illness presupposes an investigation of the

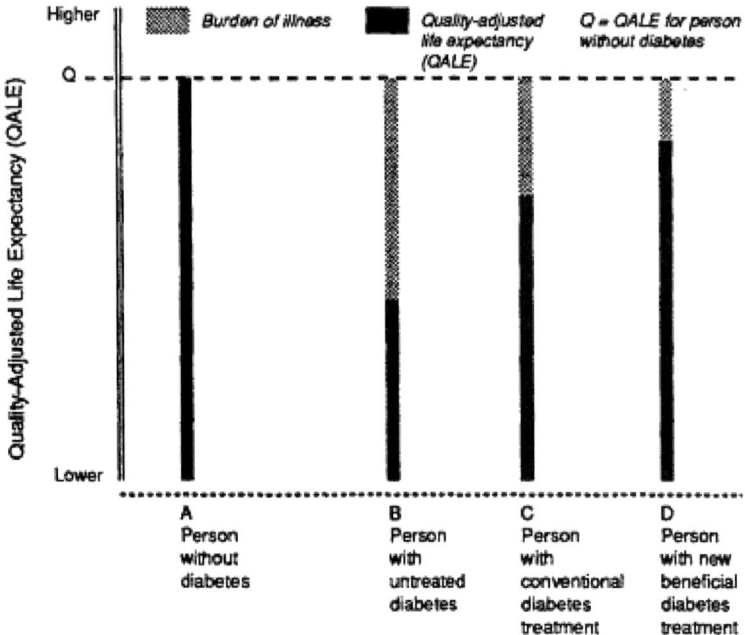

Figure 4.2 Hypothetical example of burden of illness for a person without Type II diabetes and for individuals with untreated diabetes, with conventionally treated diabetes, and with new, beneficial treatment for diabetes. Given a specific QALE for a person without diabetes, the burden of illness is seen here as the difference in quality-adjusted life expectancy for a person with diabetes treated conventionally (not an untreated diabetic) and a comparable person of similar age who does not have diabetes. If the technology to be assessed is new (e.g., continuous subcutaneous insulin), the compromise in quality of life due to diabetes would be estimated for patients managed without the new technology but with conventional technology (e.g., once-daily insulin therapy and diet); similarly, if the technology to be assessed is an established one, the QALE would include that technology (e.g., once-daily insulin therapy and diet).

technology's application to relevant clinical conditions. If the technology is appropriate for more than one condition, the burden of illness could be expressed as the sum of the burden of illness scores of the individual conditions, each weighted by the relative frequency with which the technology is used for that condition.

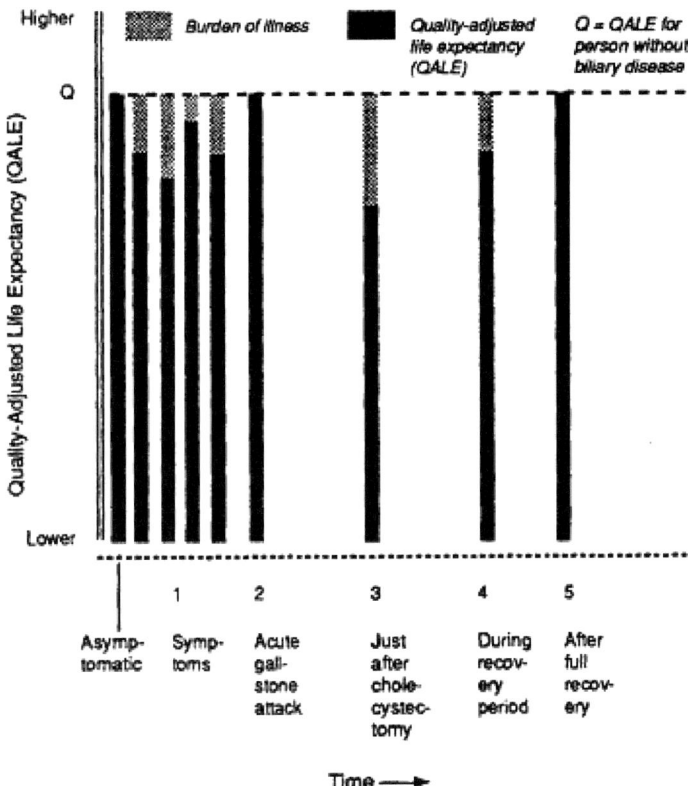

Figure 4.3 Hypothetical example of burden of illness over time for a person with asymptomatic biliary disease, acute gallstone attack, and surgically treated biliary disease. Here, the burden of illness for persons suffering from this acute condition (gallbladder disease) would include (1) measures of pain or other symptoms during a symptomatic period, (2) pain at the time of an acute gallstone attack, (3) the burden of surgery, (4) the burden of hospitalization and recovery, and (5) postrecovery. All measures are averaged over a year (or a lifetime, if that time horizon is used). The conventional treatment would be standard surgical treatment (e.g., open or laparoscopic cholecystectomy, depending on which is considered "standard").

Burden of illness here is expressed at the level of an individual patient, albeit for the "typical" patient, not as aggregate burden of illness over the entire nation. This latter is a function of another priority-setting criterion—the prevalence of the condition.

For technologies, the burden of illness is that caused by all (or the most important) conditions for which the technology is used in medical practice. For example, if the topic of assessment is computed tomography (CT) of the chest and abdomen, the change in QALE would be the sum of the changes in QALE of conditions that can be diagnosed by this type of CT scan, each weighted by the relative frequency with which the technology is used for that indication. In the case of a technology that is to be assessed for a single use, such as CT scan for gallbladder disease, the burden of illness would be the burden for gallbladder disease of patients managed without CT scans compared with patients of a similar age without gallbladder disease.

Induced Suffering. In most illnesses, the patient bears the brunt of the suffering. In illnesses such as substance abuse, however, other people are often victims of crime, assault, and motor vehicle accidents attributable to the patient. This induced suffering is important in assessing the societal importance of a clinical condition. For example, for each alcohol-involved driver who dies in a vehicle crash, other lives are lost (statistically, an additional 0.7 person dies in addition to the alcohol-involved driver; Phelps, 1988). The life-years lost for the driver count as a "direct" burden of the alcohol consumption; the life-years lost for the additional 0.7 person count as an "indirect" burden of illness and could be convened to a quality-adjusted measure of life expectancy. The committee recommends including in estimates of the burden of suffering for a clinical condition the suffering experienced by the victim of a patient's illness.

Instructions. For each condition and technology, it will be necessary to make a subjective judgment that takes into account mortality, morbidity, and health-related quality-of-life data in trying to estimate quality-adjusted life expectancy. The first step is to identify the technology with the highest burden of illness and assign it a scale score of, say, 5. The second step is to identify the technology with the lowest burden of illness and assign it a scale score of, say, 1. The third step is to assign intermediate scale values to the other listed conditions and technologies.

Data Sources. The data used to develop scores are mortality and morbidity data and health status measures, when available. Data on the loss of quality-adjusted life expectancy from all medical conditions are not sufficient to estimate burden of illness as defined by the IOM committee for all candidate topics; as a result, the panels must use surrogate measures. The Centers for Disease Control publishes information on years of productive life lost for some conditions; the IOM committee believes that extending these data to all conditions should have high priority. Because these data are not, at present, widely available, estimates are likely to be based on currently available data on mortality, morbidity, and functional status measures. For instance, Stewart and coworkers (1989) and Wells and colleagues (1989) have demonstrated health status "profiles" in terms of physical, social, and role functioning and well-being for nine chronic conditions and for depression as part of the Medical Outcomes Study. Condition- or age-specific measures have also been reported for conditions such as asthma, diabetes, and chronic obstructive pulmonary disease, for children, and for patients receiving outpatient renal dialysis (Medical Care Supplement, forthcoming); other measures are being developed by patient outcomes research teams. As health status measures become more available, this criterion will become increasingly data based.

Criterion 3: Cost

Definition: Cost is the total direct and induced cost of conventional management *per person* with the clinical condition. This definition applies to assessments of a clinical condition and to assessments of a technology.

Comments. As applied to assessing a technology, this definition presupposes an assessment of the technology's application to one specific clinical condition. If the technology is applied to more than one condition, costs are calculated as the sum of the costs of the individual conditions, each weighted by the relative frequency with which the technology is used for that condition.

Costs may be defined as annual costs or lifetime costs, depending on the time horizon, but the definition must be consistent with the definition of prevalence, as noted in the "Comments" on the preceding criterion (see also Table 4.2). The ideal solution is to use lifetime costs. In most cases, however, the lack of data on lifetime costs and the natural history of a clinical condition mean that annual costs must be used.

As defined by the committee, total cost does *not* include indirect costs, such as time lost from work because of illness or as a result of obtaining medical care. Indirect costs are not included because they are a part of the measure of burden of illness.

Total cost *does* include expected cost, which takes into account the unpredictable consequences of a clinical condition. The expected cost of an event is the product of the probability of the event and its cost. For instance, for the clinical condition "chest pain due to ischemic heart disease" (angina pectoris), the expected costs would include the possibility of suffering a myocardial infarction in addition to the known or already experienced effects of the angina. In other words, expected cost is the sum of the costs attributed to the most important of the consequences of angina pectoris weighted by the probability that each would occur.

Induced Costs. Sometimes medical conditions or events create externalities that impose costs on others. Total costs comprise the costs induced by the condition (including its impact on people other than the patient) as well as the costs directly attributable to the clinical condition. In the IOM committee's approach, the costs of such externalities should be added on a per-disease basis to direct costs just as induced burdens ("induced suffering") are added to the burdens of illness in criterion 2. These "indirect" costs and burdens are likely to occur most often for contagious diseases or for medical conditions that contribute to the occurrence of "accidents," interpersonal violence, and so forth. Costs associated with the suffering of victims of crime, assault, and motor vehicle accidents attributable to the patient are important in assessing the societal importance of a clinical condition. The committee recommends including these costs when they constitute a significant proportion of the total costs of a clinical condition.

Data Sources. Data are available from HCFA files on hospital payments aggregated by diagnostic groups and on paid and reimbursed amounts for Medicare Part B (e.g., physicians' services). Charges may also be obtained from insurance company and state data bases and from publications of the National Center for Health Statistics (e.g., *Vital and Health Statistics*). Required data, however, may not be available in the form needed or may not be available at all; new data sources may be required. The true costs of production often are not available. Because many health care delivery systems have complex accounting and financing systems that depend on discounting and cost-shifting, the use of charges must be accepted as a tenuous, but often necessary, proxy for costs. A further complication is that different organizations may not use the same accounting assumptions. Although obtaining accurate data on costs appears to be complex, the problem can and should be solved, not only for the purposes of priority setting but also for planning for health care systems of the future.

Criterion 4: Variation In Rates Of Use

Definition: Variation in rates of use is the coefficient of variation (the standard deviation divided by the mean).

Comments. The purpose of this criterion is to measure the degree of consensus about appropriate management. The premise of practice variation research is that patients are the same across the compared units. Thus, a large coefficient of variation of use rates implies a low level of consensus on appropriate management but may also reflect the availability of technology and health care financing.[5] A low level of consensus may mean that there is great benefit from doing an assessment that might lead to a higher level of consensus.

Instructions. The biggest challenge to using this criterion is to define the most relevant units for measuring variation: these might be rates of hospital admission for a condition, rates of performing a procedure for a given condition, or rates of performing a diagnostic test for a given condition.

Data Sources. For this criterion, TA program staff would assemble data on variations in per-capita use rates across different venues of care. Comparisons of per-capita use rates may be among small geographic areas, among nations, or even among different methods of paying for health care. Staff would gather the data using Medicare files, insurance company claims, or state data files. For a number of procedures and services, coefficients of variation for small geographic areas are already available in the health services research literature.

Criterion 5: Potential Of The Results Of An Assessment To Change Health Outcomes

Definition: An assessment's potential to change outcomes is the expected effect of results of the assessment on the outcome of illness for patients with the illness.

Comments. The expected effect of an assessment on patient outcomes is the probability that the assessment will affect outcomes multiplied by the magnitude of the anticipated effect. Using the expected effect takes into account both the size of an effect and the likelihood that it will occur. Panel members derive a score by estimating the probability that the assessment will lead to a change in quality-adjusted life expectancy.

The expected effect on patient health outcomes can be either beneficial or deleterious. The committee believes that the absolute value of a change,

---

[5] Although availability of technology and health care financing may contribute to variation in use rates, their contribution has not been demonstrated convincingly in the literature. For example, regional differences in insurance coverage in the United States cannot add more than about 0.02 to a coefficient of variation (Phelps, forthcoming; Phelps and Mooney, 1991). Further, variations in Britain and Canada are similar in magnitude and pattern to the United States, despite the differences in financing.

not its direction, is the important attribute when ranking a clinical condition or technology for the assessment.

Estimating this criterion is not a simple matter. When assigning a criterion score, the panel needs to take into account (1) the possible results of the assessment (will it show that one of the patient management strategies leads to a large change in outcomes?), (2) the likelihood that administrators, payers, and policymakers will use the findings for decision making, (3) the likelihood that clinicians will modify their practices, and (4) the likelihood that patients will accept the change.

Instructions. Criterion 5 is measured on a subjective 1-to-5 scale. In practice, the panel would identify the condition or technology whose assessment has the highest potential to change health outcomes and assign it a scale score of 5. Panel members would also vote on a condition or technology whose assessment has the lowest potential to change health outcomes and assign it a score of 1. TA program staff would then count the votes and identify the panel's choice of the conditions or technologies for which the results of the assessments would be most likely and least likely to affect patient outcomes. Subsequently, individual panel members would assign intermediate scale values to the other technologies, and program staff would calculate the mean scale value of each candidate topic.

Because the estimate should encompass the population for which the technology will be used, the TA staff's background briefing must specify that population. For example, for testing or screening, the population is that group to which the test is applied, not those who actually benefit. The population must be the same as the one used to estimate the burden of illness.

Data Sources. This is a subjective criterion.

Criterion 6: Potential Of The Results Of An Assessment To Change Costs

Definition: An assessment's potential to change costs is the expected effect of the results of the assessment on the costs of illness for patients with the illness.

Comments. The expected effect of the results of an assessment on costs is the probability that the results of the assessment will affect costs multiplied by the magnitude of the anticipated effect. Using the expected effect takes into account both the size of an effect and the likelihood that it will occur.

The expected effect of an assessment can be either beneficial or deleterious; that is, an assessment may lead to large decreases or to large increases in cost. The absolute value of a change, not its direction, is the important attribute when ranking a clinical condition or technology.

Instruction. Criterion scores are assigned using the method described for criterion 5.

Data Sources. This is a subjective criterion.

Criterion 7: Potential of the Results of an Assessment to Inform Ethical, Legal, and Social Issues

Definition: The potential to resolve ethical, legal, and social (ELS) issues is the probability that the results of an assessment comparing two or more conditions or technologies will help to inform an important ELS issue.

Comments. This seventh criterion gives panelists an opportunity to take a broad social perspective and to ask whether there is anything about this particular condition or technology that has not been captured in the first six criteria and that warrants an assessment. The expected effect of the results of an assessment on ethical, legal, and social issues is the probability that the assessment will affect the issues multiplied by the magnitude of the anticipated effect. The expected effect of the results of an assessment can be either beneficial or deleterious. The committee believes that the absolute value of a change, not its direction, is the important attribute when ranking a clinical condition or technology for assessment.

Instructions. Each panel member would select a scale score from 1 to 5, which would express the probability that the results of an assessment will provide information about an important ethical, legal, or social issue, multiplied by a subjective estimate of the size of the effect, if there is an effect. The committee believes that panelists will usually assign a technology or clinical condition a scale score of 1, or close to 1. It identified three categories of questions to help in estimating this criterion score:

1. "Orphan" issues. Does the panel member believe that information about the care of this condition has been retarded because this condition is relevant only to a very small number of individuals with the condition? If so, would the results of an assessment reduce this gap in information? An example might be gene therapy for a particular type of hereditary anemia. If this topic does not achieve a high priority score based on prevalence (as would surely be the case), it might still achieve high priority on the basis of the ELS criterion if the panel believes that concerns about gene therapy in general are significant.

2. Inequity. Does the panel member believe that services are inequitably distributed among persons with this condition and that this maldistribution might be reduced by information from technology assessment? For example, if a screening test is covered by private but not public insurance, would information from an assessment showing it to be very cost-effective be likely to lead to coverage by public programs?

3. Legal and legislative controversy. Does the panel member believe that an important legal or legislative controversy might alter existing clinical practice or coverage policy? If so, could the controversy be resolved through information from technology assessment? For example, a pending legal case about coverage for autologous bone marrow transplantation might be resolved by an assessment, thereby avoiding lengthy legal proceedings. In another example, if an assessment showed that breast cancer screening was not cost-effective, the assessment might lessen pressure for state legislation mandating coverage.

To assign a criterion score, each panel member would consider the ELS issues for each candidate condition or technology and determine a score as follows, depending on his or her response to the issues and questions described above:

- a score of 1 corresponds to "no" (i.e., no important ELS issues are likely to be resolved);
- a score of 5 corresponds to an intense "yes" (i.e., important ELS issues are likely to be resolved).

All panelists must have access to the same list of possible ELS issues that an assessment might resolve. A two-stage process could be used to produce such a list. In the first stage, each panelist would write down all of the ELS issues that came to mind. If the panel is actually meeting, it could discuss each issue; if the rating process is to be conducted by mail, staff would compile a list of ELS issues and send it to the panel members. In the second stage, the panelists would individually assign an ELS scale score to each condition or technology. The panel would discuss any condition for which the range of scores is greater than 2 scale points (where the range is defined as the difference between the highest and lowest score given to that condition), and panelists would have an opportunity to revise their scores. The first-round scoring can proceed quickly, as most of the conditions or technologies will be rated as 1. Discussion could be limited to those issues with a score response range of at least 2 points.

Some committee members recommended that a panelist's final ELS score for a condition or technology be the highest score given for *any* of the three categories; others preferred to use the average score. In either case, the final criterion score is the mean of all panelists' scores (either highest or average) and can range from 1 to 5.

Criteria Rejected by the Committee

The committee considered but rejected many topics as criteria for assessment or reassessment. Two bear special mention because of their inclusion in the IOM/CHCT pilot study. The first—likely enhancement of national capacity for technology assessment—is a useful and desirable secondary effect, but the committee did not consider it central to priority setting. The second—the availability of sufficient data to complete the assessment— seems at first to be a reasonable criterion. However, the committee believes that if a condition merits assessment on the basis of other factors, the response to lack of data ought to be to set in motion some process that would yield the needed data (see further discussion of this issue in Chapter 5). The one exception might be a technology that is too new to be assessed.

Step 6. Computing Priority Scores

The sixth element of the IOM process is calculation of priority scores. Once criterion scores and weights are assembled, the priority score for each condition or technology can be computed by combining the objective and subjective criterion scores. Priority scores for each condition or technology are derived from the data for the objective criteria and the scale scores for the subjective ratings, each adjusted by the weight given to each criterion. Once priority scores have been calculated, TA program staff list the candidate technologies and conditions in the order of their priority scores. Higher scores will be associated with conditions and technologies of higher priority.

The formula for calculating the priority score is the sum of the natural logarithms of the criterion score weighted by the importance of the criterion. The formula for a priority score for condition or technology j, then, is:

$$\text{Priority Score}_j = W_{1j}\ln S_{1j} + W_{2j}\ln W_{2j} + \ldots + W_{7j}\ln S_{7j} = \sum_{i=7}^{k} W_i \ln S_i \quad (2)$$

or their mathematically equivalent forms,

$$PS = S_1^{W_1} S_2^{W_2} \ldots S_7^{W_7} = \prod_{i=1}^{7} S_i^{W_i} \quad (3)$$

where W is the weight for each criterion described in Step 1 of this process. Two illustrative calculations are shown in Table 4.4. Priority scores for the

Table 4.4 Calculation of Two Examples of the Priority Score

		Example 1: Cardiac Condition		Example 2: Acute Surgical Procedure	
Criterion	Criterion Weight (W)	Criterion Score (S)	W(lnS)	Criterion Score (S)	W(lnS)
Prevalence	1.6	30[a]	5.44	100[a]	7.37
Burden of illness	2.25	4.3	3.28	1.7	1.19
Cost	1.5	9,000[b]	13.66	1,800[b]	11.24
Variation in use rates[c]	1.2	0.36	-1.23	0.17	-2.13
Potential of the results of assessment to change health outcomes	2.0	3.2	2.33	3.7	2.62
Potential of the results of assessment to change costs	1.5	4	2.08	2	1.04
Potential of the results of an assessment to inform ELS issues	1.0	2.0	.69	1	0
Priority score			26.25		21.34

[a] Number/1,000 in U.S. general population.
[b] Annual cost (in dollars) per year.
[c] Coefficient of variation.

entire list of candidate topics are easily calculated with a spreadsheet program, using as input the mean criterion scores.

One can convert the log-additive model to the multiplicative model by taking the antilog, that is,

$$PS = \exp(\ln(PS)), \qquad (4)$$

where $\exp^y$ equals e raised to the y power.

Derivation of the Model

As shown above, the multiplicative model becomes additive when one takes the logarithm of it. The committee adopted a multiplicative model for priority setting because such models exhibit a number of desirable characteristics in comparison with additive models. In multiplicative models, both the rank order and relative size of the priority scores of various medical interventions are preserved regardless of the scale of measurement of the criterion scores. Thus, for example, it does not matter whether prevalence is measured in cases per 1,000 or cases per 100,000 in the general population, as long as the same unit of measurement is used for every technology and condition being assessed. (A shift from measuring prevalence in cases per 1,000 to cases per 100,000 would cause that particular criterion score to fall by a factor of 100 for every intervention; the overall priority score for every intervention would fall by 100 raised to the power of the relevant criterion weight [e.g., 1, 0.5, 2, or whatever weight had been applied to that criterion score in the model]). Such changes shift the magnitude of every score by an equal amount, and hence do not alter ranks or relative sizes of scores. The change is similar to counting the size of the national debt in dollars, pennies, or billions of dollars; the units of measurement do not change the actual size of the debt.

Similarly, in terms of the subjective components of the priority system (e.g., the ELS score), it will not matter whether the minimum score can be 0.01, 0.5, 1, 10, or some other number; as long as all scores are set relative to the smallest score used, the relative ranking is preserved. Thus, a criterion with a weight of 1 should be defined as twice as important as a criterion with a weight of 0.5 in the same way that a criterion with a weight of 2 should be twice as important as a criterion with a weight of 1. The magnitude of the minimum ELS score is immaterial as long as the ELS panel consistently assigns criterion scores for other conditions and technologies relative to the smallest score assigned. Appendix 4.2 to this chapter discusses scaling and transformation issues in more detail.

Readers will observe that the formula for calculating the priority score corresponds to the conventional understanding of the social impact of disease, which is seen as the product of the number of people with the illness times the burden per person times the cost per person, and so forth. Moreover, as the committee recognized and as is seen in Table 4.4, prevalence and cost, because they are expressed as real rates rather than as subjective scores, may tend to dominate the final value for the priority score unless higher weights are given to the other criteria.

In sum, the model yields a constant *relative* rank ordering regardless of the units in which the criterion scores are expressed. The same is true for the magnitude of the priority score for a condition or technology relative to all others. Table 4.5 illustrates this point using a model with two criteria, cost and prevalence, applied to three conditions (A, B, and C).

Determining Whether Assessment is Desirable and Feasible

The next step in the priority-setting process is to decide whether a highly ranked candidate topic should be assessed by OHTA and whether enough information exists to perform the assessment. Two circumstances would argue for deferring technology assessment for a given condition or technology despite a high priority score: (1) another organization with a record of performing rigorous and credible assessments has recently completed or has an assessment under way; and (2) there is insufficient high-quality clinical and scientific information about the technology to conduct an assessment. One important task for OHTA staff will be to obtain information

Table 4.5 Example of Priority Scores Obtained Using Prevalence Expressed as Cases per 1,000 and per 100,000 Persons in the General Population

Condition	Unit Cost	Cases/1,000 Persons/Year		Cases/100,000 Persons/Year	
		Prevalence	Priority Score	Prevalence	Priority Score
A	$100	1	9.2	100	23.0
B	$100	10	16.1	1,000	29.9
C	$100	100	23.0	10,000	36.8

Note: In this example, all three conditions have the same unit cost ($100) but differ in prevalence. If one applies a model with two criteria (cost and prevalence) to three conditions (A, B, and C), and assigns a weight of 2 to unit cost and a weight of 3 to prevalence, the priority score would be calculated as below:

Priority Score = $2 \ln S_{cost} + 3 \ln S_{prevalence}$

where S is the criterion score.

about the activities of other organizations that do technology assessment. Obtaining such information will require some form of network through which organizations can share information about their current activities. Familiarity with the published literature is another important responsibility of OHTA staff and will require searching the literature for relevant material and evaluating the usefulness of such articles.

When the information on which to base an assessment is too weak to support it, OHTA might choose to issue an interim statement to the effect that data are unavailable for assessment of the condition or technology. One function of such a statement would be to call for action (e.g., funding for extramural research) to eliminate the information gap.

Indeed, the committee urges that all candidates for assessment be assigned priority scores, even when the staff or panels realize at an early stage in the priority-setting process that the data for an assessment are not available, because a high priority score for a candidate could help to shape the nation's research agenda. This discussion is continued in Chapter 5.

Step 7. Review by Ahcpr National Advisory Council

The seventh and final element of the IOM priority-setting process is review. The IOM committee recommends that there be independent, broad-based oversight of the priority-setting process, preferably through the AHCPR National Advisory Council. After taking the council's advice into account, the administrator of AHCPR would publish a list of the agency's priorities for assessing medical technology.

The purpose of the AHCPR National Advisory Council is to advise the Secretary of Health and Human Services and the Administrator of AHCPR; it includes "making recommendations to the Administrator regarding priorities for a national agenda and a strategy for (A) the conduct of research, demonstration projects, and evaluations..." (Public Law 101-239, SEC 921,b,2,A). The Council meets three times a year. Apart from ex-officio members, it includes eight individuals distinguished in the conduct of research, demonstrations, and evaluations; three from the field of medicine; two from the health professions; two from business, law, ethics, economics, or public policy; and two representing the interests of consumers of health care. The legislation also calls for establishment of a subcouncil (the Subcouncil on Outcomes Research and Guideline Development); currently, an additional subcouncil on general health services research and technology assessment functions as well.

The AHCPR National Advisory Council has authority to review and recommend adjustment of the results of peer review study sections that review grant proposals for extramural research funding; it can raise the standing of a grant proposal that does not score high enough to receive funding. Reviewing and, if warranted, recommending the adjustment of priority rankings for technology assessment would be an analogous function in the sphere of OHTA's work.

This committee recommends that the AHCPR National Advisory Council be involved in review of the results of the priority-setting process. A major outcome of such involvement would be to lend credibility and political support to the priority-setting process. The council could perform other functions as well. For example, it could group the priority scores into categories, such as "most important to assess," "very important to assess," and "low priority for assessment." Within these categories, appropriate designations can indicate items that were borderline in terms of the group into which they fell. This form of categorization according to priority score would allow a "softening" of the numerical priority score to prevent the process from being seen as more precise than it actually is. After reviewing the priority list, the AHCPR Council could, on the basis of its own deliberations, recommend changes in the priority ranking of individual items in the interests of balance—for example, balancing technologies that are chiefly used for one age or for another demographic group; balancing interventions for preventive, diagnostic, and therapeutic procedures; or balancing technologies used in various settings of care.

Similarly, the Secretary of Health and Human Services and the AHCPR administrator may need to preempt the process or adjust the priority rankings. There may be rare circumstances in which the national interest will dictate that the priority-setting process be set aside for the sake of a compelling issue of public importance that the formal criteria do not capture. Building these functions of the council, administrator, and secretary into the priority-setting process is an important precaution against too mechanized an approach. A balance needs to be maintained between a systematic, logical, tamper-proof process and an approach that is flexible enough to have credibility and to serve the national interest when circumstances so dictate.

REASSESSMENT

Role of Reassessment in the Complete Assessment Program

Is the process of assessing a technology or condition for the first time different from the process of reassessing a topic that has been *previously* considered? The committee believes that these processes should be fundamentally similar. Moreover, for OHTA at least, a single budget allocation covers evaluation of health technology—whether for the first time or as a reassessment. Therefore, the committee recommends that only one process for setting priorities for technology assessment be invoked.

Operationalizing this process means that conditions and technologies that have never been assessed by OHTA will compete for priority with topics that OHTA assessed at an earlier time. The panel should apply the same priority-setting criteria to candidates for a first-time assessment and candidates for reassessment. The committee also believes, however, that OHTA has a special obligation to consider previously assessed topics as candidates for re-evaluation. There are several reasons for this view.

First, and foremost, OHTA assessments (although not formal recommendations to the Health Care Financing Administration, or HCFA) are a matter of public record. These assessments may carry considerable weight among payers, physicians, and even patients. Therefore, it is important that these opinions reflect current knowledge. If more recently available information might invalidate an earlier OHTA recommendation, OHTA must decide whether it is necessary to reconsider the evidence by reassessing the condition or technology. For instance, one or more newly published journal articles may contain information that sheds new light on the performance of a previously assessed technology, or a study of a new, competing technology may appear in the literature. Another impetus for reassessment might be the occurrence of a serious epidemic that raises the prevalence of a disease to the point where guidance for using a technology may require revision (Box 4.1)

Second, OHTA may itself acquire advance knowledge of information that might lead it to consider reassessment. For instance, during a first-time

---

Box 4.1 Events That Might Trigger Reassessment

- A change in the incidence of a disorder (or its prevalence, if the condition is chronic) or in the degree of infectiousness of a biological agent
- A change in professional knowledge or clinical practice, including a recent rapid change in utilization and increased variability in the use of a given technology
- Publication of new information about a technology that suggests a change in its performance or cost
- The introduction of a new competing technology
- A proposal to expand the use of the treatment to populations not included in the original assessment (e.g., expanding breast cancer screening to women aged 40 to 49 when earlier work focused only on women aged 50 and older)
- Publication by another organization of a high-quality, conflicting assessment.

assessment, OHTA may know that circumstances are likely to change within some reasonable, known time frame and that that change would warrant a consideration of reassessment. Similarly, OHTA may be aware that pivotal clinical trials or effectiveness studies are under way or about to be started, or staff may learn of new technologies that are being tested outside government circles. Alternatively, AHCPR may provide funding for studies (e.g., the Patient Outcomes Research Team investigations) to generate new knowledge, perhaps on topics that had been brought into the foreground initially by an OHTA assessment.

Third, for OHTA, conducting a reassessment may be more efficient than performing an initial assessment. Both the method and process used in an initial assessment may still be applicable, and many of the original data sources may still be useful. In these circumstances, the greater ease and lower cost of a reassessment may make it an attractive choice and may raise its priority standing.

Fourth, because a topic cannot be reassessed unless it has received a high enough priority score to warrant a first-time assessment, topics that are chosen for reassessment are likely to be important by definition.

In sum, although previously assessed technologies and conditions should compete for available assessment monies on fundamentally the same criteria that are used to determine first-time assessments, the committee concluded that OHTA has an obligation explicitly to consider previously examined topics.

Methods of Identifying Candidates for Reassessment

The IOM committee recommends a four-step process for considering a previously assessed topic for reassessment (Figure 4.4): (1) tracking of topics of prior assessments, (2) evaluation of the quality of those studies that suggest that reassessment might be needed, (3) panel review to decide if changes in a given technology or clinical practice seem to warrant reassessment, and (4) placement of the topic on the candidate list for ranking with candidates for first-time assessment.

Ongoing Tracking of Events Related to Previously Assessed Topics

Stated Time of Review for First-time Assessments. Both at the time of an initial and of a subsequent assessment, OHTA should explicitly state whether a reassessment is likely to be needed and when it expects that circumstance to occur. Early reassessment might be necessary in fields that are changing rapidly or when a clinical trial is completed. Often, however, OHTA will assess relatively stable, mature technologies. When setting priorities, OHTA should informally review all previously assessed conditions and technolo gies and decide whether newly emerging information about any topic might indicate a need for reassessment.

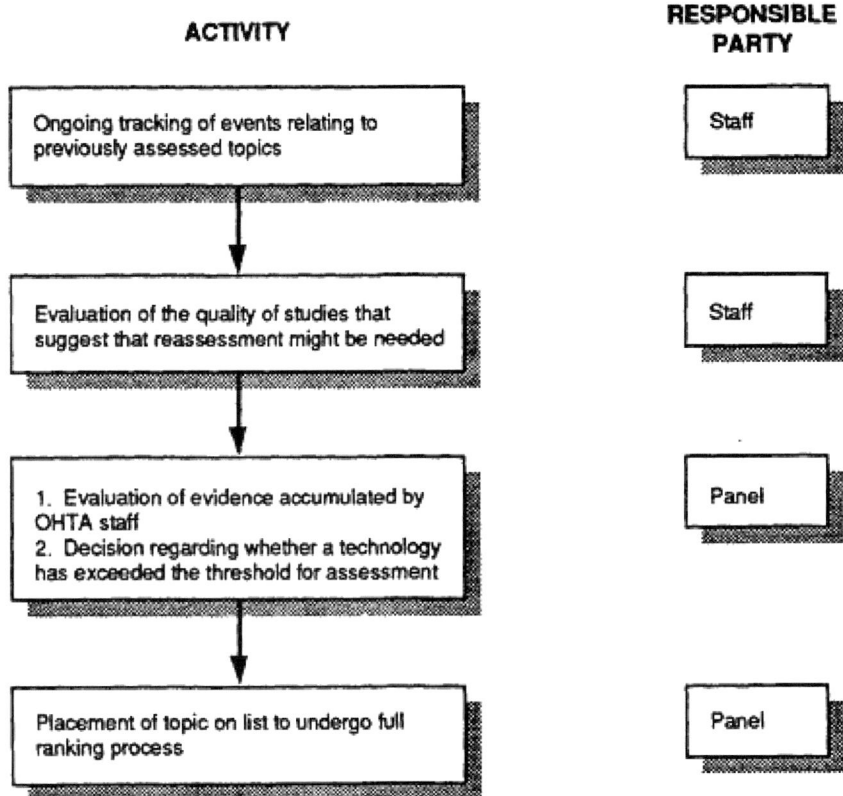

Figure 4.4 Proposed process for reassessment.

Catalog of First-time Assessments. OHTA currently provides information about its assessments in individual *Health Technology Assessment Reports*. To document events that might apply to previously assessed topics, the committee strongly recommends that OHTA create a separate catalog of its previous assessments, keep it current, and cross-reference it by conditions and technologies. The catalog should include specific characteristics for each assessment, such as

- the disease condition studied;
- the intervention(s) studied;
- the population to which the assessment applies (similar to entry criteria for a randomized controlled trial);

- the methods used in the study;
- types and sources of data (e.g., claims data from Medicare, randomized controlled trial data from the literature);
- the dates of collection of the study's data and of the study report;
- indications of how much an assessment has been used (e.g., changes in financing policy, citations in medical journals); and, when feasible,
- evidence of effects on clinical practice.

The catalog is the starting point for tracking technologies that have been previously assessed. Ideally, a public agency would also track assessments by other organizations, and OHTA is a logical repository for these data. Such a task might also be undertaken by the National Library of Medicine.

Monitoring the Published Literature on Previously Assessed Topics. The agency should establish a system to monitor the published literature on previously assessed topics, given that up-to-date knowledge of a topic is the foundation for reassessment. Using the search strategies of the original assessment, the staff should monitor the literature to identify high-quality studies that could have a bearing on the decision to reassess and the occurrence, if any, of one of the triggering events listed in Box 4.1.

OHTA might also consider creating a network of expert consultants or seeking the support of medical specialty groups who would take responsibility for monitoring the literature on a topic and calling attention to developments that might warrant OHTA reassessment. The IOM has made recommendations for augmenting information resources on health technology assessment in two recent reports (IOM, 1989b, 1991b).

Evaluation of the Quality of Studies

Once literature regarding a topic has accumulated, OHTA staff should evaluate the quality of the studies. Additionally, experts in the content and methodology of the clinical evaluative sciences could review designated studies to advise OHTA on the quality of the evidence being presented. The agency could then decide whether a reassessment is desirable—that is, whether events have occurred since the first assessment that have rendered the original conclusions obsolete. An OHTA panel, presumably a subpanel of OHTA's priority-setting panel, should periodically review the data on previous assessments and decide whether the circumstances warrant reassessment.

Ranking Candidates for Reassessment

The committee recommends that candidates for reassessment be considered on the same basis as candidates for first-time assessment, using the same process. Thus, OHTA panels would consider topics for first-time assessment at the same time that they consider topics for reassessment, and OHTA would forward one list of candidates for assessment (or reassessment) to the AHCPR Advisory Council. That list would have both candidates for first-time assessment and candidates for reassessment. Figure 4.5 shows the interrelationship of the process for first-time assessments and the process for reassessment.

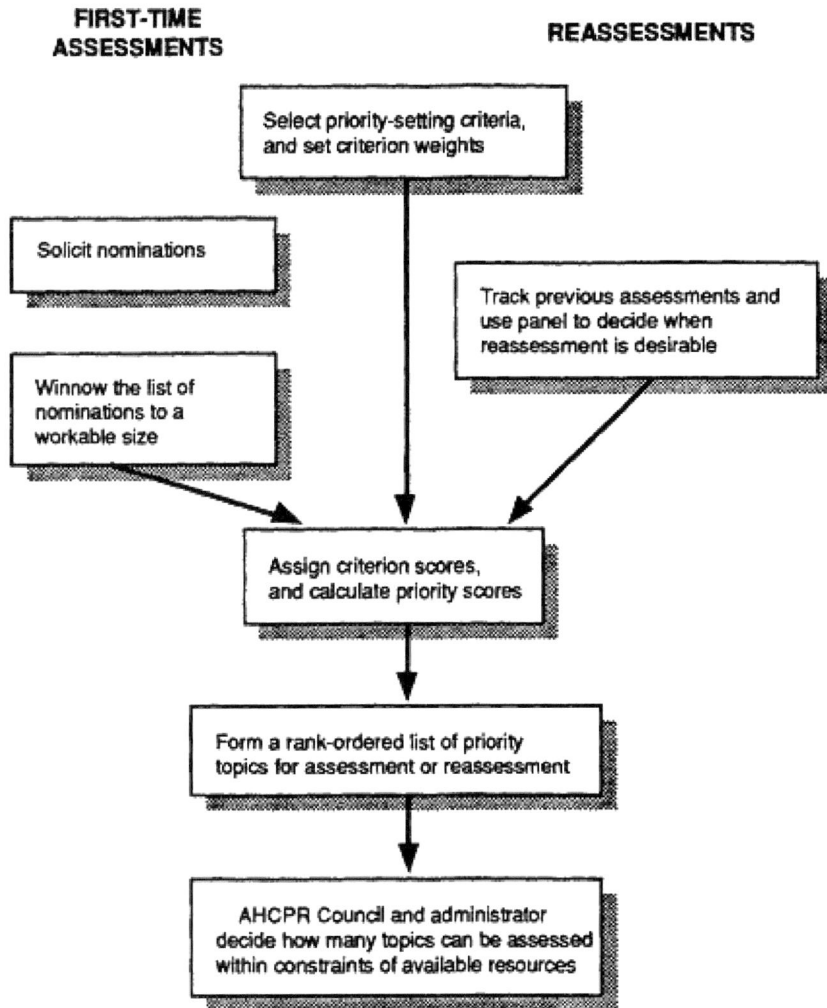

Figure 4.5 Relationship between process for first-time assessment and process for reassessment.

Final Steps after Establishing Priority for Reassessment

After calculating priority scores for reassessment candidates, OHTA should address two additional pertinent topics: the results of a sensitivity analysis and the cost of reassessment.

Sensitivity Analysis

If a previously assessed topic has achieved a high priority score, OHTA staff should use the data that have been assembled for setting criterion scores to perform a sensitivity analysis. The purpose of the analysis is to test whether the new information would change the conclusions of a previous assessment. For example, if a diagnostic device (technology A) was assessed previously and a new device that is potentially more accurate but that will cost $300 more per patient has become available, a simple sensitivity analysis might indicate whether the recommendations about the use of technology A would change. If those recommendations would not change, even if technology B had perfect sensitivity and specificity, there would be no reason to conduct an assessment of these technologies—not, at least, until the cost of technology B falls relative to technology A.

Cost Analysis

The cost of reassessment will vary widely. Some reassessments will be simple and relatively inexpensive to perform; others will require almost a complete rethinking of the problem. For instance, some analyses, such as those using decision-tree formats, easily permit reassessment as data change. If a new randomized trial alters the perceived treatment effect of an intervention, one can readily incorporate the new data in such an analysis and re-estimate the cost-effectiveness of various interventions included in the tree. Other reassessments, however, may require a more fundamental change in the analytic approach or incorporation of an entirely new measure of outcomes or costs.

SUMMARY

The committee has proposed a priority-setting process that includes seven elements: (1) selecting and weighting criteria for establishing priorities, (2) eliciting broad input for candidate conditions and technologies; (3) winnowing the number of topics; (4) gathering the data needed to assign a score for each priority-setting criterion for each topic; (5) assigning criterion scores to each topic, using objective data for some criteria and a rating scale anchored by low- and high-priority topics for subjective criteria; (6) calculating priority scores for each condition or technology arid ranking the topics in order of priority; and (7) requesting review by the AHCPR National Advisory Council. The chapter defined the seven criteria and explained how to assign scores for each one. Three of the criteria—prevalence, cost, and clinical practice variations—are objective; they are scored using quantitative data to the extent possible. The other four—burden of illness and the likelihood that the results of the assessment will affect health outcomes, costs, and ethical, legal, and social issues—are subjective; they are scored according to ratings on a scale from 1 to 5.

The chapter also addressed special aspects of priority setting that apply only to reassessment of previously assessed technologies; these include recognizing events that trigger reassessment (e.g., change in the nature of the condition, in knowledge, in clinical practice); the need to track information related to previous assessments; and the obligation to update a previous assessment as a fiduciary responsibility and to preserve the credibility of the assessing organization.

APPENDIX 4.1: WINNOWING PROCESSES

This appendix discusses in greater detail some of the issues that arise in reducing a long list of candidate conditions and technologies (or "winnowing") for possible assessment by the Office of Health Technology Assessment (OHTA). Three general methods are discussed as a basis for the winnowing process: (1) eliciting some sense of the intensity of preference regarding a candidate on the list on the part of those who nominate it and using this information to winnow; (2) using a single criterion and a process similar to but much simpler than the quantitative model; and (3) using an implicit, panel-based process. The appendix offers options within each method and provides a rationale for the committee's suggested choices.

Intensity Rankings by Nominating Persons and Organizations

One difficulty with the "open" nomination process is that it does not necessarily reveal the intensity of the preferences of nominating individuals and organizations. Thus, one way to help establish preliminary priorities is to request nominators to include a measure of intensity and then to add these measures of interest across all nominating organizations and persons, using the final total as a preliminary ranking. Several variants on this approach are available:

- *Option A*. Ask each nominating group to assign a rank from 1 to 5 (1 = least important; 5 = most important). If an item is not mentioned on a ballot, it receives a rank of 0.) Sum the ranks across all ballots. Using that

figure as a preliminary ranking, proceed to final ranking on (for example) the top 50 candidates.
- *Option B.* Proceed as in Option A but allow each ballot to have a fictitious budget of $1,000 to allocate across all candidate technologies. TA program staff would then add the budget allocations across ballots. For example, an organization could specify $4 for 250 technologies and conditions, $250 to only 4 technologies, or $1,000 to a single technology. This process has the desirable feature of reflecting the scarcity of research resources available for technology assessment.
- *Option C.* Use a more formal "willingness to pay" (WTP) revelation process familiar to economists (e.g., "Clark taxes"). Such techniques attempt to measure directly the willingness of an organization or person to pay for the assessment of a specific technology. The aggregate willingness to pay for a technology assessment (summed across all ballots) represents a measure of the social value of the assessment. (Indeed, some people would assert that, if a WTP assessment is properly done, it could be used as the final priority-setting list.) The committee does not believe that enough is known about the actual conduct and reliability of Clark tax-type methods to base current priority-setting methods on this approach alone, but some organizations may find this technique useful at least in a preliminary stage.

Overall, the committee believes that the use of methods like these for preliminary priority setting—at least in pure form—*within the context of a public agency* creates some important problems. Its questions center on the issue of who is eligible to submit "ballots" and how much each of those ballots should "count." For example, if open submissions of ballots are allowed or welcomed, and each has equal weight, then lobbying organizations could readily "stuff" the ballot-box with numerous ballots, each emphasizing a single technology. (All-Star baseball voting exhibits some of this characteristic, in that fans in some cities may try to tilt the balance in favor of players on their home teams.)

One alternative is to limit the distribution of ballots or to determine in advance how much each ballot counts. (For example, the ballot of a large health insurer might count much more than that of an individual provider, and the ballot of a single-purpose charity devoted to the cure of a single disease might reflect some estimate of the size of its constituency.) However, a preliminary assignment process of this kind inherently opens up the entire process to intense political pressure, and, indeed, makes it likely that the process will become so expensive that it loses its value as a low-cost screening device.

"Open" voting with specified preference intensity (i.e., option A) raises the possibility that private interests with a strong interest in having a single technology evaluated might spend considerable resources to bring this about. The importance of OHTA assessments in some Medicare coverage decisions is an obvious reason for attempts to control the priority-setting process.

Yet in other settings, these intensity-based preference systems might function extremely well. For example, an association of primary care physicians or a large health maintenance organization (HMO) might wish to undertake its own technology assessment activities and establish its own priorities for this activity. In this case, the membership of the society, the staff, or enrollees of the HMO form a natural basis for voting, and there would be no presumed preference on the part of any one person in these groups to have any single technology evaluated—except as it might affect the well-being of patients. For this reason, the committee includes a description of these preference-intensity voting systems, but it cautions against their use in settings in which they invite strategic responses.

Preliminary Ranking Processes

The winnowing process uses (initially) one criterion from the final ranking system (e.g., prevalence of disease, disease burden, cost per treatment, variability in use) and provides an initial ranking on that basis. This method is more data intensive than the first set of winnowing methods described above but less data intensive than a complete ranking. There are two main variants on this idea:

- *Option D*. Rank all nominations on the criterion that receives the highest weight in the final priority-setting process, keep (say) the top 250, and rank those, using both the highest- and second-highest-weight criteria. This list becomes, in effect, a restricted version of the final ranking process. Keep (for example) the top 100 candidates, and conduct a full ranking on that set. The logic of this approach is that the criterion weighted highest will in many ways determine the final ranking; at least, it must be true that nominations receiving a low score on the highest-ranked criterion cannot ever receive a high enough score to make a "final 20" or some comparable list. This hierarchical approach thus eliminates nonviable candidate technologies, at a lower data-gathering cost than a complete ranking of each technology, while preserving the essential features of the ranking system.
- *Option E*. In the preliminary ranking, one could select the criterion to be used in the initial ranking according to not only the weight assigned in the process but also the costs of data gathering. For example, if the highest-weighted criterion had very high data-gathering costs but the next-highest-weighted criterion had much lower data costs associated with it, one could conduct the initial ranking using the second-highest-weighted criterion instead of the highest-weighted criterion.

These types of preliminary ranking systems have an obvious disadvantage: they require that data be collected on a potentially large number of technologies. This reason alone may argue against their use in a setting where a widespread "call" to suggest interventions is likely to produce a large number of candidate topics.

Another, more subtle issue deserves mention: using other methods for preliminary screening produces an independence between two parts of the priority-setting system that the use of only one technique cannot achieve. Some people may view as a virtue the idea that the winnowing system and the final ranking system follow the same methodological basis. Others may see this commonality as a defect to be guarded against by using an alternative method for preliminary screening.

Panel-Based Preliminary Weighting

On balance, the committee believes that methods from a third group of options are preferable for preliminary screening. This approach uses one or more panels of experts to provide preliminary (subjective) rankings of the nominated technologies. To minimize costs, these activities could be conducted using mail ballots, or (a modern variant) electronic mail. Two principal versions of this process are possible:

- *Option F. Double-Delphi system.* Use two separate panels, constituted with quite different memberships, and have them select (say) their top 150 technologies (and leave them unranked). Keep for final priority setting only those technologies that appear on both lists. As an alternative, each panel could "keep" perhaps 50 technologies, and the final ranked list would include those that appeared on at least one list. The Delphi rankings could be based either on subjective, implicit judgments of panel members (which makes this tactic a relatively low-cost alternative) or on data supplied to the Delphi panels (a higher-cost option). The two Delphi panels should have distinctly different memberships; in one case, perhaps, the panel would be entirely health care practitioners, and in the other, health services researchers, consumer representatives, and others not directly involved in providing care. Particularly if no data were to be presented, it would be necessary to have panels that possessed sufficient technical expertise to understand the implications of their decisions.
- *Option G. Single-panel in-and-out system.* This approach would use only a single expert panel that would generate two sets of technology lists. The topics on the first list (consisting, for instance, of 5 percent of the submitted nominations) would automatically go forward to the next step in the process. The bottom (say) 50 percent of nominations would be excluded from further consideration. The remaining 45 percent (in this example)

would go to a second-tier winnowing process. The second-tier process could be either (a) a repeat of this process or (b) some sort of data-driven system similar to option D above. This process is entirely self-contained if used recursively. As an example of such a "recursive" use, let us suppose that the original round of nominations had produced 800 candidate technologies for evaluation. During the first round, 5 percent (40 technologies) would be retained and 50 percent (400 technologies) would be eliminated from consideration, leaving 360 technologies. Reapplying the same rules but keeping (for example) 10 percent during this round and eliminating (again) 50 percent would retain 36 and eliminate another 180 technologies, making a total of 76 technologies preserved at this stage and 144 as yet unclassified. Finally, keeping 10 percent of these unclassified technologies would bring the total to 90, and the process could stop there. These 90 technologies would continue through the full priority-setting process.

Comment

The final choice of a winnowing method for an organization could well depend on the degree of openness rather than the expert knowledge desired in the process. The most open systems are those in the first group discussed earlier (options A-C) because they rely on intensity of preferences as expressed by nominating organizations. Because of their openness, however, they intrinsically invite expenditure of private resources and attempts to control the system. The third group of approaches (options F and G) makes fullest use of expert knowledge. The second set—ranking on the basis of a subset of the eventual criteria—best preserves the intent of the final priority-setting process but is more data intensive and thus potentially more costly. Organizations engaged in priority setting may also find it useful to use a winnowing process that quite deliberately *does not* use the same approach as the final process. They would then use activities from the first or third groups rather than the second.

As was argued earlier, because of the intrinsic problems associated with the first two groups of winnowing strategies as applied in the OHTA setting, the committee recommends that OHTA adopt as a preliminary winnowing system either options F or G in the panel-based set. The committee has no strong preference for either option; ease of implementation thus could be a key consideration in the ultimate choice. Option G offers a recursive system on the grounds that it is easier to pick "the top" and "the bottom" of any list than it is to rank every element within it.

In other settings, the other methods have potential value and may well be preferred to any from the third group. For example, in settings with a narrow focus that leads to a limited number of submissions, dam-driven methods similar to those in the second group (options D and E) may be the best, particularly if the organization conducting the priority assessment values consistency of method in the preliminary and final priority-setting process. In other arenas, options from the first group (A, B, and C) may have considerable appeal, particularly for those with a naturally closed population from which nominations might emerge and in which no particularly strong stake exists in having any single technology or condition studied. Finally, one can imagine combinations of the processes; for instance, a panel-based preliminary ranking might use options B or C to distribute votes or hypothetical dollars.

Regardless of the choice of process, the committee believes that it is desirable in any priority-setting process to rely at least in part on nominating organizations to provide information relevant to the final process—for example, information on costs, prevalence of disease, burden of disease, and variability of treatment use across geographic regions.

Finally, it must be remembered that the winnowing process plays only a minor role in determining the eventual set of activities chosen for technology assessment. Its only goal is to speed up (and reduce the costs of) the final priority-setting process. To the extent that winnowing achieves this goal at low cost and without eliminating technologies that would otherwise be assigned high priority, it has succeeded; conversely, to the extent it becomes elaborate and expensive, it defeats the purpose of using any winnowing strategy. For these reasons, the committee advises the choice of a winnowing technique that reflects the goals of simplicity, avoidance of control by special interests, and low cost.[6]

APPENDIX 4.2: METHODOLOGIC ISSUES

Two key methodologic issues for deriving a formula for the technology assessment priority score are (1) the scale on which each of the criterion scores is expressed and (2) the means used to maintain consistent relationships among the weights assigned to each criterion. In regard to scaling, the priority-setting process outlined by the committee uses logarithms of each criterion score. The discussion that follows explains the choice of the particular logarithmic approach used by the committee.

The IOM priority-setting process uses "natural" units for objective criteria, such as the prevalence of a condition and the costs of care for the condition (e.g., "head counts" for the number of affected, dollars for cost).

---

[6] Low cost in this context includes both public and private expenditures. Procedures established within the priority-setting process that invite considerable investment by private parties to manipulate them are self-defeating.

Yet, one approach, using natural units would mean that every weight could be affected by a change in the scale of any other measure. For example, a quite natural scale of measurement of per-capita spending is the proportion of spending on the disease that is related to the range of spending on all diseases under consideration. Thus, if per-capita spending ranged from $1 per person (at the low end) to $1,000 (at the high end), one could use a measure of where $500 fits between the low and the high end (i.e., 500/(1,000 - 1) = 500/999 = 0.5), rather than the $500 itself. With this type of measure (scaled by the *range* across all interventions), the value for the criterion score would be 0.5. In a model based on natural units, to maintain the importance of "spending," one would have to modify the *weight* so that the product of the criterion weight and the criterion score remained unchanged. Thus, if the scale of measurement of any of these components were changed, the weight would also have to be changed to keep the product unchanged.

The problem of the interaction of the weights and the scale of measurement of the values that determine a criterion score can be avoided by a simple mathematical modification. By using *relative importance* to determine the criterion weights, the logarithmic transformation provides the same results independent of the scale by which each of the component "scales" is measured.

Properties of Logarithms

For those not familiar with the mathematics of logarithms, it may be helpful to review two of their properties. In the general equation $b^y = x$, the exponent y is called the log of x to the base b (one can describe the log as the exponent y to which the base b must be raised to get number x). Thus, an equivalent expression is $y = \log_b x$.

The first property of logarithms is that $\log_b (xw) = \log_b x + \log_b w$. That is, the log of the *product* of x and w is the sum of the log of x and the log of w (thus, we use the term "multiplicative" or "log additive" to describe the committee's model).

The committee's model might use a logarithm with any base, but the committee chose to use natural logarithms (ln) in which the base is e (an irrational number whose decimal expression is 2.71832 ...). Substituting the term ln for log and the expressions S_1 and S_2 for x and w, respectively, it is apparent that $y = \ln S_1 + \ln S_2$.

The second property of logarithms helps to explain the role of criterion weights: $\log_b (x^r) = r \log_b x$. In other words, raising the log of x to the power r is equivalent to multiplying r by the log of x. Again, substituting the committee's expressions as above shows that raising the log of the criterion score to the weight for that criterion is equivalent to multiplying the criterion weight by the natural log of the criterion score. Thus, y = Priority Score, and, as in Chapter 4, Equation (1) is as follows:

$$\text{Priority Score} = W_1 \ln S_1 + W_2 \ln S_2 + \ldots + W_7 \ln S_7 \qquad (1)$$

Application to the Iom Model

The use of logarithms is neither intuitive nor familiar to most people, but it does express a natural way of thinking. The logarithmic transformation will accomplish the desired scaling, no matter what "natural" scaling is used. All that is necessary to implement this approach is for participants in the priority-setting process to agree that the relative weights represent the *relative importance* of a criterion. One can then measure the individual score components in any way one desires, as long as measurements are consistent across technologies for a criterion. Weights of 1 yield proportional increases in priority as a component increases. Weights of 2 increase a priority score 20 percent for each 10 percent increase in a criterion score.

To provide an example of how use of relative importance can eliminate worry about how the various components in the criterion scores are measured, let us consider the Phelps and Parente (1990) model. In this model, N = number of people treated annually, P = average cost per procedure performed, Q = average per-capita quantity, COV = the coefficient of variation for the procedure across regions, and e = the demand elasticity. The priority-setting index I for intervention j is:

$$I_j = N_j P_j Q_j COV^2_j / e_j \qquad (5)$$

If one assigns the relative importance weights for each element in Equation (5) as 1, 1, 1, 2, and -1 and takes the logarithm of each, then

$$\ln(I_j) = \ln(N_j) + \ln(P_j) + \ln(Q_j) + 2\ln(COV_j) - \ln(e_j) \qquad (6)$$

Mathematically, the effect of changing the values of the variables on the right side of Equations (5) and (6) can be expressed in terms of percentages. Thus, a 10 percent increase in the number of people treated for intervention j (N_j) raises the value of I_j by 10 percent (and similarly for P_j and Q_j); a 10 percent increase in the COV_j increases the index by 20 percent; and a 10 percent increase in e_j decreases the index by 10 percent.

Using logarithms is an approach that is intended to reflect relative place on a scale of importance. In producing priority scores for each candidate condition or technology, the relative *ranking* of each procedure will be the same, regardless of how each of the criterion scores is measured. The relative *difference* in priority scores similarly will be unaffected by changes in the scale used to measure any criterion score.

5

Implementation Issues

The Institute of Medicine study committee believes that the priority-setting process presented in Chapter 4 would be valuable to and is feasible for use by all organizations engaged in health technology assessment—not just the Office of Health Technology Assessment (OHTA) of the Agency for Health Care Policy and Research (AHCPR). Both the compilation of the data that are needed for the priority-setting process and a list of priorities created through a national, broadly representative process would be useful to many technology assessment programs.

This chapter describes how the process proposed in Chapter 4 serves several objectives. First is the need for broad-based input in setting criterion weights and in developing subjective criterion scores for priority setting so that the weights and scores reflect societal preferences. Second is the need for professional expertise to integrate diverse scientific data, to adjudicate when data conflict, and to provide a base of experience from which to estimate missing data. Third is the need for an efficient process that can be carried out at a reasonable cost. This chapter describes how to implement the priority-setting process, suggests a cycle for priority setting, and estimates the resources that would be needed to set priorities for health technology assessment and reassessment.

THE PRIORITY-SETTING CYCLE

The priority-setting cycle comprises the steps listed below performed according to the time frames indicated.

Repeat every 5 years or more infrequently:

- Set criterion weights (this step requires a panel, as discussed below).

Repeat at least every 3 years:

- Solicit nominations of candidate conditions and technologies.
- Reduce the list of nominations through the "winnowing" procedure laid out in Chapter 4 and Appendix 4.1.
- Obtain the data required for the objective criteria.
- Review the objective data and decide what will be used to calculate the priority score (this step requires a panel). Establish the subjective criterion scores (this step requires a panel).
- Calculate the priority score.

The next section presents key points about setting criterion weights. Later, the chapter discusses critical concerns regarding the remaining activities in the context of resources needed to implement the process and, more specifically, the responsibilities of the priority-setting panel.

SETTING CRITERION WEIGHTS

The criterion weights mentioned above in the priority-setting cycle and examined in Chapter 4 are intended to represent the preferences of society. The committee envisions a broadly constituted panel that would set criterion weights not oftener than every 5 years. Once OHTA has established the weight-setting system, it should test and establish its reliability; then it could repeat the procedure only infrequently. Although the committee sees this weighting task as a group process, it might be accomplished by some other means (e.g., voting by mail), if those means were shown to be reliable. Although AHCPR's National Advisory Council might function as this weight-setting panel, the committee suggests that a separate group be constituted for this and subsequent panel tasks, in part because the task requires a particular array of expertise, but also because the workload could be considerable.

Apart from setting the criteria weights, the committee sees the priority-setting cycle as occurring every 2 to 3 years, but not less frequently than every 3 years, because of the current pace of technological change. The time that elapses before repeating the process would depend not on a fixed interval but on how many assessments have been completed.

The number of assessments—as opposed to the number of conditions and technologies that the quantitative model can rank—will depend principally on staff resources for data collection and secondarily on the experience of the panels in generating criterion scores. As a rule of thumb, the committee suggests that the quantitative model should rank three to four times the number of conditions and technologies that are likely to be assessed in a given cycle. This would allow other organizations to use the list to select topics for technology assessment.

RESOURCES NEEDED TO IMPLEMENT THE PROCESS

The resources needed to implement the process are the technology assessment (TA) program staff and the weight and priority-setting panels. Both are discussed below.

Technology Assessment Program Staff Requirements

The committee carefully considered the resource and staffing requirements entailed by the process described in Chapter 4 from two perspectives: the current constraints on OHTA and AHCPR and the (idealized) goals of a credible, sound, defensible model process. This priority-setting process, based on the committee's experience with the pilot test, will require resources. However, the resources required to implement the ideal version of this committee's process may not be available, given the current budget and staffing levels of OHTA. The committee viewed its report, in part, as setting reasonable goals for the agency and for OHTA. Therefore, the following detailed discussion of program resources is appropriate for an optimum program rather than a minimum program.

The process will require enough staff to accomplish its mission of allocating the country's technology assessment resources wisely. The committee views the priority-setting process as a public good that will be one of OHTA's most valued products, and it recommends that the agency provide sufficient staff to generate priority rankings that will be useful not only for its purpose but for other organizations that also perform technology assessment. During the process of compiling data for the quantitative model, OHTA will create a valuable data base (containing, for example, such information as cost per case for the top 50-ranked disease conditions), which will itself be a resource to other organizations. A further benefit of the data base will be that once information on candidate conditions and technologies accumulates, later iterations of priority setting are likely to be less expensive.

The committee believes that implementing a process such as the one suggested in this report requires staffing that is at least comparable to that for a grant review study section: a mid- or senior-level, analytically trained scientist who is well grounded in health services research; one or two junior to mid-level staff; and clerical support. Staff responsibilities would include the following:

- Conduct regular literature searches to maintain information about conditions and technologies that have been assessed previously.
- Convene and manage the panels.
- Solicit nominations of candidate conditions and technologies for assessment and reassessment.
- Compile data on the frequency of conditions, the costs associated with their care, and variations in practice patterns.
- Draft summary documents for the panels to use in assigning scores for each criterion of the quantitative model. During the committee's pilot test of the quantitative model, one full-time-equivalent staff person took a day to assemble the data for one condition; by that metric, over the course of a year, one staff person could probably assemble data for about 200 conditions.
- After the panel has generated priority rankings, staff would also conduct informal surveys of other professional and assessment organizations to determine whether any of the conditions and technologies being considered for assessment by OHTA are already being evaluated.

Because the quantitative model requires information on seven aspects of each candidate condition or technology, the number of program staff will determine the number of conditions that will be ranked. The process of reducing the list of nominations to a number that is within the staff's capacity—the "winnowing" of the list—is relatively crude. A number of options for such winnowing are discussed in Chapter 4 and its Appendix 4.1. However, a general rule of thumb should be kept in mind: the "cruder" this preliminary winnowing process is, the more likely it will be that important technologies are mistakenly omitted from the final list.

Priority-Setting Panel

To understand the tasks of the priority-setting panel, it is helpful to refer to Figure 4.1, which showed the steps and participants for the proposed model. Specifically, the priority-setting panel has four primary tasks, as listed below. As noted earlier, task 1 occurs approximately once every 5 years, and tasks 2-4 occur about once every 3 years.

Task 1: Select criteria and set criterion weights.
Task 2: Reduce the long list of candidate conditions and technologies to a more manageable size (i.e., "winnowing").
Task 3: Generate subjective criterion scores.
Task 4: Generate objective criterion scores.

The committee recommends that OHTA convene a single "standing" panel to perform all of these tasks. The panel could be organized like a research study section: panel members thus would serve rotating, staggered 3-year terms. Staggered membership is important to sustain an institutional memory about the conceptual details of the priority-setting system. The committee sees the panel as a broadly representative standing committee with individuals who represent a balance of perspectives and who have "front-line" knowledge of health care as providers, patients, and third-party payers. Thus, it will require individuals with expertise in the following areas: medicine and surgery, nursing, social work, health economics, epidemiology, health care statistics and health demography, law, bioethics, health administration, health technology manufacturing, employee health benefits, and health insurance. The committee also advises that the panel include one or more patient and consumer representatives. Most, if not all, members of the main panel should have sufficient knowledge of clinical conditions and technologies (for instance, to be able to generate scores for the subjective criteria, as in task 4). Some, but not all, members will need the quantitative and medical knowledge to be able to make informed quantitative estimates for objective criteria (as in task 3).

For the first task—defining criteria and assigning criterion weights (see above)—the panel would be brought together and function as a "plenary" group. For other tasks, as explained below, it might be divided into more specialized subpanels. Depending on the eventual workload or the needed perspectives and expertise, or both, additional persons might be appointed to one or another of the subpanels. The discussion that follows, however, is couched in terms of all subpanels being constituted with individuals from the main standing group. It is also assumed that members of the main panel might well serve on more than one subpanel.

For task 2—winnowing the larger list of topics to produce the final set of candidates toward which the remaining priority-setting activities are directed—the committee believes that more than one subpanel might be created from the original panel. Generally, for this task, the subpanel(s) should be as broadly representative as possible—within the constraints that arise from dividing up the main panel.

Tasks 3 and 4—developing the criterion scores for the subjective and objective criteria, respectively—might also be performed by subpanels created from the main panel. Here, the assignments to subpanels might be more along "expert" lines, with groups for the subjective criteria being more "broadly representative" and those for the objective criteria being more "quantitatively expert." The latter subpanels, for instance, require individuals with quantitative reasoning skills and epidemiologic expertise to adjudicate among conflicting data and estimate prevalence, costs, illness burdens, and practice variations in cases where data are missing.

The workload of the subpanels, and therefore the number of subpanels, will depend on the number of conditions or technologies under consideration. If, for tasks 3 and 4, the workload requires more than one of each type of subpanel (as proposed above), the subpanels can divide their assignments. In this case, the committee recommends that each subpanel work with every topic and assign a subset of the criterion scores rather than take a limited number of topics and assign a score for each criterion. This approach would ensure that the subpanel is consistent across all topics when it assigns the scores for a given criterion.

IMPLEMENTATION CONSIDERATIONS FOR OHTA AND OTHER ORGANIZATIONS

The foregoing discussion addressed the tasks and resources necessary to implement the committee's proposed priority-setting process. During implementation itself, OHTA must resolve several additional issues, including the following:

1. Establishing the validity and reliability of the priority-setting process and its various elements. The committee believes that OHTA (as well as other professional organizations that may employ this suggested process) has an obligation to examine its validity and reliability.
2. Altering the definitions and weights of criteria—points to keep in mind during this effort.
3. Developing a strategy for cases in which the data necessary to develop criterion scores are missing (a separate problem from lack of data to conduct an assessment, which is addressed separately below).
4. Determining the kind of product or products that the priority-setting process should yield.

Validity and Reliability

How can OHTA validate a process that is based in part on subjective judgment and prediction? The concept of "validity," in the sense of the "correct," "true," or "gold standard" does not seem entirely suitable to priority setting. It would be appropriate, however, to determine the usefulness, appropriateness, or cost-effectiveness of the results of the process, holding that adoption of the process is evidence of acceptability, feasibility, and generalizability.

One can ask whether the process seems reasonable to people who are familiar with either priority setting, technology assessment, or the technologies themselves. This mechanism would gauge what is sometimes called *face validity*. Another aspect of face validity is whether the process is, in fact, used and considered useful by the group for which it is intended (i.e., OHTA) and by other groups.

A priority-setting process is *reliable* if the same group produces the same (or similar) rankings at different times or if a different group (or subgroup), whether constituted similarly or quite differently, produces similar results when given exactly the same information and instructions. Reliability could be tested readily for parts of the process (e.g., criteria weighting, estimation of data for an objective criterion, ratings for a subjective criterion) and for the entire process. The use of systematic sampling frames and sufficiently large groups would allow standard statistical tests of reliability.

Criteria

Choosing—and Changing—Criteria

After extended discussion, the committee selected seven criteria by which to implement its principles of priority setting; these were described in Chapter 4. The criteria encompass the current social impact of a condition for which a technology is used, variations in use rates, and the likely changes that an assessment would engender. Further, because a simple listing of criteria would be insufficient to consistently implement the process proposed by the committee, the criteria have been carefully defined so that they can be used dependably in a quantitative model. Their reliability, however, under different conditions of use, must be established through field testing.

Other organizations may wish to augment or change the criteria or their definitions. When doing so, it is important to understand several features of the seven criteria being proposed in this report. First, in terms of social impact, the criteria are symmetrical with respect to current health and economic burden and expected change in health outcome and cost as a result of the assessment. Burden of illness and cost are considered separately as valid social and economic aspects of illness. Because they are considered separately, they can, and might be expected to be, given different weights by different organizations.

Second, impact of illness is commonly viewed as the product of burden of illness and prevalence. This formulation treats as equivalent a large burden of illness borne by a few individuals and a small burden of illness borne by many persons. Different weights given to each criterion, however, can express social attitudes about such mathematical equivalence. Further, a low prevalence score can, to a degree, be counteracted by a high score for the criterion concerning ethical, legal, and social issues. This balancing might occur in instances in which the priority-setting panel has special concerns about the assessment of a technology used for a small, defined patient population whose illness might not otherwise have sufficient leverage to attain a high priority score.

Third, the criteria do not assume that a given direction of change (e.g., higher or lower cost, improved or worsened health outcome) raises (or lowers) the assessment priority of a condition or technology. Although the direction of change may be of considerable concern in doing assessments, the magnitude, not the direction, of change is important in setting priorities. Those choosing technologies for assessment are presumed to be equally interested in whether, for instance, a technology is likely to cause a large rise or an equally large decrease in expenditures.

Criterion Weights

During its pilot test, the committee designated weights (see Appendix A, Figure A.1) for the priority-setting criteria in its process; in this effort, it attempted to use the perspective of a public agency. The committee considers these weights merely illustrative and recognizes that a given organization would probably wish to derive its own weights for priority setting.

Availability of Data to Generate Criterion Scores

The priority-setting process recommended by the committee requires the use of data in explicit ways. However, the committee is well aware of the limitations of published data for use in generating criterion scores. Prevalence and mortality data are not necessarily available at the level of specificity needed; additional problems are that they may include only subpopulations such as the elderly and may be confounded by severity and case mix. Moreover, cost estimates inevitably will not include all costs, and aggregate data on functioning and well-being are scant.

Nevertheless, the committee argues that the priority-setting process should proceed with whatever data *are* available. It should also use the best estimates it can generate for resolving conflicting or missing data. Further, it should encourage the development of better epidemiological data bases. In this sense, the distinction that is drawn between subjective and objective criteria is a matter of degree.

For instance, the criterion "burden of illness" must at present be considered largely subjective. Yet if the high weight given this criterion by the pilot test is replicated by other groups, this would argue strongly for greatly improved data on health outcomes for untreated and "conventionally" treated illnesses (see Ellwood, 1988).

Publicly Available Products

The committee envisions two products from the OHTA priority-setting process that would be publicly available: a listing of the priority-ranked technologies and the data base used to construct it. In addition, both products would form the basis of a priority-setting document to be published by OHTA. The list might include all technologies, even those that were winnowed out, or it might include only those that remained after winnowing to which the quantitative model was applied. The list might include specific priority rankings as an indication of the distance between a given technology and the next highest (or lowest) ranked technology, or it might simply group the technologies. As noted earlier, grouping the technologies in the final product would help to avoid a false sense of precision.

The committee is strongly in favor of an open priority-setting process. To that end, it believes that the priority-setting document should include rankings and selected summary data that contributed to the criterion scores of each technology. Each highly ranked technology should also be accompanied by a discussion of the features of the technology that were considered in its ranking, a description of the data sources that were used, and a discussion of the level of confidence that the panels assigned to these data (the strength of the scientific evidence). Calling for such documentation is consistent with recommendations from another IOM committee concerned with the appropriate development and implementation of clinical practice guidelines (IOM, 1990c, forthcoming).

The data base available to the public would include the weights assigned to each criterion and the objective and subjective criterion scores for each condition and technology to which the quantitative model was applied. Such a data base would be useful not only to OHTA but to other organizations that wished to set priorities. It can be challenged, corrected, and amplified by researchers, specialists, and disease-oriented interest groups; and it might well act as a stimulus to better data acquisition. Both functions are consistent with the goals of AHCPR in promoting the public good through improved information about health care.

In a formalized process, such as the one proposed in this report, an important consideration is how to acknowledge and include strongly held minority views and, if needed, stimulate further data development. The committee recommends that each time a substantial or strongly held minority view is voiced by members of the panel, the document include those views either in a "discussion section" or in a section immediately following the discussion of the majority view. The inclusion of such opinions would be especially important later during reevaluation or reassessment because they would alert TA program staff to specific events or evidence that might prompt reassessment.

WHEN THE SCIENTIFIC EVIDENCE IS INSUFFICIENT FOR ASSESSMENT

Often, a topic has high priority for assessment but insufficient evidence to support the assessment activity. In such circumstances, the committee believes that OHTA's appropriate response is to recommend a first-time assessment. Taken together, these statements (high priority, lack of data) would be a logical basis for the development of an AHCPR technology assessment research agenda. This concept, linking priority setting, assessment of the evidence, and a research agenda, is an important component for the future of technology assessment and for further enhancement of evidence-based medical practice.

Other responses to insufficient evidence—for example, an interim conditional statement or a decision-analytic model—are also possible. Given that data will always be inadequate, in some sense, the presence or absence of information does not affect *whether* but *how* a technology assessment should be done. In some cases, literature synthesis will be possible; in others, AHCPR may decide to fund secondary data analysis or primary data collection. It should be recognized, however, that the cost of generating such data may be significant.

Interim Statements

When the topic is of high priority but insufficient data are available for an assessment, OHTA might consider an analysis that would begin with the question, What level of effectiveness is necessary for this technology to be cost-effective? The congressional Office of Technology Assessment (OTA) took this approach to assess pneumococcal vaccine before the clinical trials to measure its efficacy had been completed. Because OTA did not know whether vaccine immunity would last for 8 years or a lifetime, its estimates had wide ranges of uncertainty. Nevertheless, the agency's assessment was sufficiently convincing that it led to a recommendation that Medicare cover pneumococcal vaccine.

Modeling

Assessments using decision-analytic modeling techniques to estimate expected costs and the effectiveness of alternative management strategies can be useful to simulate missing empirical data. In place of such data, the model uses expert subjective estimates of probabilities and outcomes. Analysts then employ sensitivity analysis to determine which clinical factors could cause the currently preferred alternative to be superseded by another management strategy. Later research that includes primary data collection can measure the true value of these "sensitive" variables and provide an empirical basis for further policy recommendations.

Using decision modeling to focus the attention of clinical investigators on the most important variables for decision making is a powerful concept.

For example, one assessment organization did such an assessment of the automatic implantable defibrillator when there were not enough data to conduct a cost-effectiveness analysis (Kuppermann et al., 1990). Using efficacy data and clinical studies from the literature, a panel of electrophysiologists simulated the clinical outcomes and the cost for a hypothetical cohort of patients that received the defibrillator and compared them with another cohort that did not receive the device. The estimated cost per life-year saved, using the new device as it was configured in 1986, was about $17,000. The analysts also estimated costs and effectiveness of expected updated versions of the defibrillator as it was expected to perform in 1991. In another effort, the federal government funded a separate project to collect primary data over a 3-year period. Both of these approaches are legitimate technology assessments, and both are useful responses to a lack of data. The decision modeling effort provided timely analysis using uncertain data; the empirical study will use much more valid and reliable data in a much less timely manner at a much higher cost.

In sum, empirical data from reliable published sources are currently required to conduct an assessment because OHTA conducts only literature-based assessments. This requirement presupposes that the technology has been available long enough to have been evaluated empirically. However, the armamentarium of technology assessment includes other approaches such as those described—decision modeling, other forms of estimation, analyses of administrative data sets, such as that available in the Medicare files, and interim statements—that OHTA (or other programs in AHCPR) should consider using.

SUMMARY

The committee envisions priority setting as occurring in a cycle. The panel sets criterion weights approximately every 5 years. The priority-setting cycle itself repeats at least once every 3 years and leads to a rank-ordered list of conditions and technologies. The priority-setting cycle begins and ends with involvement of persons and institutions outside the federal government. At the beginning, OHTA asks a broad range of persons and institutions to nominate conditions and technologies that they wish to see assessed. Then, OHTA staff collect the data required to set objective criterion scores and convene panels to assign criterion scores to each condition or technology. Staffing for this OHTA priority-setting activity is likely to require a level comparable to AHCPR study sections: a mid-career or senior-level professional, several junior to mid-level research staff, and clerical staff.

A broadly representative panel would be established to help set criterion weights, to reduce the list of nominations of conditions or technologies, and to assign criterion scores to each of these topics. Separately constituted subpanels might also be required to divide the workload and to assign subjective or objective criterion scores. The subpanel(s) assigning *subjective* criterion scores would be composed of individuals with the range of perspectives of the full panel; the subpanel(s) assigning *objective* criterion scores would require experts in epidemiology and health statistics to review the data collected by OHTA staff and produce estimates when necessary.

The committee envisions two products that would be publicly available: a list of the priority-ranked technologies and the data base used to construct the list. Both would be part of a priority-setting document published by OHTA. Each highly ranked technology should also be accompanied by a discussion of the features that contributed to its ranking, the data sources that were used, the level of confidence the panels assigned to the data, and any strongly held minority views.

OHTA should adopt methods that will enable it to conduct preliminary assessments even when there is not yet adequate evidence on which to base a strong clinical policy recommendation. The committee advocates using decision analysis as a way to identify which missing evidence is most important for decision making and to use the results as input to the development of an agenda for empirical research sponsored by AHCPR.

6

Recommendations and Conclusions

This committee was charged to propose a process for setting priorities for technology assessment for use by the Office of Health Technology Assessment (OHTA) (in the Agency for Health Care Policy and Research—AHCPR) and by other assessment organizations. In responding to this charge, the committee organized its work—and this report—at three levels of specification: general principles, a proposed process, and information about how to implement the process within OHTA and in other organizations that conduct health technology assessment.

This chapter has three main parts. First, it reviews the main points of the report: the rationale for the process developed by the committee, 11 recommendations (details are given in Chapters 3, 4, and 5), seven steps or tasks needed to implement the proposed process, anticipated resources and periodicity of the process, and issues that might arise during implementation.

Second, it examines how the proposed priority-setting process might be used or adapted by other organizations and for purposes other than technology assessment. Third, it discusses the committee's views on some potential problems that may arise.

REVIEW OF THE COMMITTEE'S RATIONALE AND RECOMMENDATIONS

At the outset of its work, the committee reviewed the priority-setting processes of a number of organizations. From this review, it established a set of principles to govern priority setting in a public agency such as OHTA. The *basic principle* is that OHTA's process should be consistent with its mission of directing its resources for technology assessment toward medical conditions and technologies that have the greatest impact on the well-being of the public and on the public's expenditures for health care. By adhering to this principle, the committee believes that OHTA can identify and evaluate the medical conditions and technologies whose assessment will offer maximum benefits to the nation's citizens.

Several specific benefits of an OHTA priority-setting process include the potential to improve the health and well-being of the public, reduce needless or inappropriate health expenditures, reduce inequities and maldistribution of health care, and inform ethical, legal, and social issues related to candidate topics. The committee enunciated three other objectives of a priority-setting process: it must (1) meet the information needs of users, (2) be efficient, and (3) be sensitive to the assessing organization's political, economic, and social constraints and be—as well as appear to be—objective and fair. A process that satisfies these principles and objectives is summarized in the 11 recommendations that follow.

Recommendations

Recommendation 1

OHTA should adopt a systematic process to assist decision making about which medical conditions and technologies it should assess or reassess. The process should involve a broad spectrum of interested parties and should be open to public view, resistant to control by special interests, and clearly understandable.

The process proposed by the committee would be conducted in two phases: (1) setting weights for criteria, which would be performed approximately every 5 years, and (2) implementing the rest of the priority-setting process, which would be performed approximately every 3 years.

Recommendation 2

OHTA technology assessment, whenever feasible, should focus on a clinical problem (e.g., diagnosis of coronary artery disease) rather than on a technology per se (e.g.. exercise thallium radionuclide scan). Similarly, priority setting should address clinical conditions.

Although concern about a new test or treatment often leads to calls for its assessment, whenever possible, a technology should be evaluated within the context of the clinical condition for which it is being used. There are two reasons for proposing this orientation. First, technology assessment should be comparative, implying that it should answer a useful *clinical* question: Which technology should a practitioner use and under what clinical circumstances? Second, a technology can only be evaluated in the context of what it does, which is to help solve a clinical problem.

Recommendation 3

OHTA technology assessments should compare the alternative technologies for managing a clinical condition. Similarly, the priority-setting process should include alternative technologies for managing a clinical condition.

The data required to determine the assessment priority of a clinical condition depend on which technologies are relevant to its management. (For example, the expected cost of managing a condition depends on the costs of the individual technologies that might be used.) This recommendation holds true even when a new technology is the first to be applied to a clinical problem: there are no obvious comparative *technologies*, but watchful waiting without therapeutic intervention is always a valid, and important, alternative.

Many parties need information about alternative technologies for managing a condition. For instance, clinicians and patients must choose among alternative tests and treatments. Third parties, too, are concerned about the marginal effects of a technology—the additional benefits and risks represented by one technology in comparison with another. All such comparisons should take place on a "level playing field"; that is, the same methods and clinical circumstances should be applied to all of the technologies. An analogy to empirical studies is apt: the use of historical controls rather than concomitant controls in primary research is normally not sufficient because conditions change over time and variables other than the one being singled out for study may be responsible for observed differences. The same reasoning holds for technology assessment: referring to analysis done 10 years earlier is not acceptable as a form of comparison because the techniques, methods, and assumptions of the earlier analysis may not be the same as those currently used.

Although comparative data are preferred, they are sometimes difficult to acquire—particularly in the case of many alternative approaches to a particular condition. Thus, it may at times be necessary to conduct more limited assessments.

Recommendation 4

OHTA should identify criteria that best characterize a topic's importance as a candidate for assessment. The committee recommends the following *objective criteria*:

- prevalence of the specific condition;
- unit cost of the technologies commonly used to manage the condition (or the unit cost of a technology and its alternatives); and
- variation in the rate of use of a technology for managing the condition (or variations in the rates of use of the technology and its alternatives).

Ordinarily, the data required to characterize a candidate topic may be found in the published literature or elsewhere in the public record. *Prevalence* is the number of people with the condition per 1,000 persons in the general population. *Unit cost* is the total direct and induced cost of conventional management for a person with the clinical condition. *Variation in rates of use* across different settings of care is measured by the coefficient of variation. A high coefficient of variation frequently implies a low level of consensus about clinical management.

The committee also recommends the following *subjective criteria*:

- **burden of illness imposed by the clinical condition;**
- **potential of the results of the assessment to change health outcomes;**
- **potential of the results of the assessment to change costs; and**
- **potential of the results of the assessment to inform ethical, legal, or social issues.**

Although some objective data about these criteria may exist, integration of these data often requires subjective estimates as well as judgments about the likely effect of an assessment; thus, the committee considers these four criteria subjective. Each criterion is described briefly below and is discussed in greater detail in Chapter 4.

Burden of illness, which is estimated at the level of the patient rather than of society, is the difference between the quality-adjusted life expectancy (QALE) of a patient who has the condition and who receives conventional treatment and the QALE of a person of the same age who does not have the condition. The potential of the results of the assessment to *change health outcomes* is the expected effect of the result of the assessment on health outcomes for patients with the illness. It includes consideration of the findings of the assessment and of the likelihood of policy and administrative changes, clinical practice changes, and patient acceptance. The potential of the results of an assessment to *change costs* is the expected effect of the results of an assessment on the costs of illness for patients with the illness. It includes direct costs to the patient and induced costs.

The committee anticipates that most conditions will be adequately ranked based on the first six criteria listed above. The seventh criterion, which considers the likelihood that the assessment would help to *inform ethical, legal, and social issues*, gives the panelists the opportunity to take a broad social perspective and to ask whether there is anything that had not been captured in the first six criteria that would alter the assessment priority of this particular topic.

Recommendation 5

OHTA should use an explicit process to determine a candidate topic's priority ranking. In the ranking process, the criteria that are important in deciding whether to do an assessment determine a topic's priority rank.

The committee recommends the use of a process that can be examined, challenged, and adjusted on the basis of tests of its reliability and validity. Use of a quantitative model as part of this process allows assumptions to be explicitly stated and individually assessed; it also permits the use of data, whenever they are available.

Recommendation 6

The committee recommends a specific quantitative method to calculate a priority score for each candidate topic, using the following formula:

$$\text{Priority Score} = W_1 \ln S_1 + W_2 \ln S_2 + \ldots + W_7 \ln S_7$$

where W is the criterion weight, S is the criterion score, and in is the natural logarithm of the criterion scores.

A panel of people from a broad spectrum of interests should set the criterion weights.

In the process proposed by the committee, a broadly based panel would be created to lead the necessary activities. Its first task would be to establish the criterion weights through one of several possible procedures (see Chapter 4). Once established, these criterion weights remain constant for the entire priority-setting process (i.e., across all candidate topics).

A topic's priority score determines its priority rank. According to the committee's method, each candidate topic receives a criterion score for each of the seven criteria (for example, S_1 might be prevalence expressed as a number per 1,000 persons in the general population). In addition, each criterion has a criterion weight that reflects its importance in determining priorities for technology assessment. (W_1, for example, might be a weight of 2 for prevalence, relative to a burden-of-illness criterion weight of 3.)

Each candidate *topic* has its own combination of criterion scores (S_n) for the seven attributes. The panel noted above (or a subset of its members) reviews data prepared for each topic by OHTA staff and assigns the criterion scores. Objective criterion scores are determined by a subpanel with expertise in clinical epidemiology and statistics. Subjective criterion scores are determined by a broadly representative panel (or subpanel) with expertise in health care.

The rationale for taking the natural logarithm of the criterion score is to avoid the intractable problem of combining numbers that represent attributes with different units into a summary score. The logarithm of a number solves this problem because it is unitless.

Recommendation 7

OHTA should actively solicit nominations of topics to be considered for assessment. The solicitation should include payers, health professionals and their representative organizations, manufacturers of medical products, business, labor, government agencies, and consumers of health care.

The committee judged that a widespread solicitation of topics is crucial to the success of the priority-setting effort. In particular, the solicitation should be broad enough to ensure that important technologies are not omitted inadvertently from consideration and that all important constituencies are included in the process.

Recommendation 8

OHTA should develop a structured procedure for reducing the number of nominations.

The initial number of nominations will almost certainly far exceed staff capacity to collect the data required to assign criterion scores to each topic. Therefore, the committee proposes that a formal procedure be adopted to reduce that initial list to a manageable size—a technique it calls "winnowing." To be feasible, the winnowing technique should be much less costly than the full ranking system. Practical approaches include preliminary ranking according to one or two of the objective criteria or a consensus process in which several groups would subjectively rank subsets of candidates by mail ballot.

Recommendation 9

OHTA should consider all previously assessed topics as candidates for reassessment.

OHTA has a special obligation as an influential public agency to revisit any previously assessed topics whose recommendations may be based on outdated or now erroneous information. A change in the nature of the condition, expanded professional knowledge, a shift in clinical practice, or publication of a new, conflicting assessment might trigger consideration of a condition and technology for reassessment.

Recommendation 10

OHTA should maintain a data base on each topic that has been previously assessed and should catalog information pertaining to the topic.

A catalog will make it easier for OHTA to know when to consider topics for reassessment and when newly published information is relevant to a topic that has been previously assessed. Information should include descriptions of data, populations, and methods used in the earlier assessment, the impact and controversy generated, and a topic-specific estimated date or interval for considering reassessment.

Recommendation 11

OHTA should set priorities among topics for reassessment at the same time and on the same footing that it sets priorities for first-time assessment. That is, the committee recommends that OHTA create one rank-ordered list that contains both topics for reassessment and topics for first-time assessment.

The process of determining the need for reassessment can be accommodated within a priority-setting process for first-time assessments with the addition of several specific components: (1) a system for tracking previous assessments and events that prompt recognition that a major factor (e.g., a clinical condition or practice, information) has changed relative to the old assessment; (2) evaluation of literature that suggests that reassessment might be needed; (3) a decision by the priority-setting panel that a technology or clinical practice has changed sufficiently to warrant reassessment; and (4) a sensitivity analysis that suggests that the conclusion of an initial assessment might change when a reassessment is conducted.

There are several steps in deciding to do a reassessment. The first is to decide whether events that have occurred since the first assessment have made the original conclusions obsolete, as outlined in recommendation 10. The second step in reassessment is to evaluate the quality of studies that suggest that assessment might be needed. Third, an OHTA panel, presumably a sub-panel of OHTA's priority-setting panel, should periodically review the data on previous assessments and decide whether the circumstances warrant reassessment.

Fourth, topics designated for reassessment would be added to the list of candidates for first-time assessment that survive the winnowing process.

If a previously assessed topic has achieved a high priority score for reassessment, program staff should use the data that have been assembled for setting criterion scores to perform a sensitivity analysis. This analysis would indicate whether the new information would change the conclusions of a previous assessment. If a sensitivity analysis indicates that current recommendations about the use of a technology would not change, even given the reasons for a reassessment, no reassessment should be undertaken.

REVIEW OF STEPS AND ISSUES IN IMPLEMENTATION

The committee has proposed seven steps for its priority-setting process. Each step, which is explained in greater detail in Chapter 4, is summarized below. Also discussed in Chapter 5 and summarized below are four implementation issues: the resources needed for implementation of the process, how often priority setting should occur, what products of the process should be available to the public, and what should be done when there is insufficient evidence to conduct an assessment based on a review of the literature.

Steps in a Priority-Setting Process

Step 1. Selecting and Weighting the Criteria Used to Establish Priority Scores

This step requires that a broadly representative panel be constituted to select and define the criteria to be used for priority setting. In recommendation 4 and in Chapter 4 of this report, the committee defined seven criteria and recommended that they be adopted for use by OHTA. Chapter 5 discussed a number of points to be considered before changing the criteria or their definitions. In addition to selecting and defining criteria, the panel noted above would assign each criterion a weight that reflected its relative societal importance.

Step 2. Identifying Candidate Conditions and Technologies

OHTA program staff would seek nominations from a wide range of groups concerned with the health of the public. This solicitation is likely to produce a large set of candidate topics.

Step 3. Winnowing the List of Candidate Conditions and Technologies

Earlier in the report, the committee described several methods to reduce (winnow) the set of candidate conditions. The committee suggests one particular method—a so-called panel-based preliminary ranking system—that is less data intensive than the other methods, but also less costly than the full ranking system, free of bias, resistant to control by special interests, and easily understandable to all participants. The method uses one or more panels to provide preliminary (subjective) rankings of the nominated technologies. To minimize costs, these activities could be conducted using mailed ballots.

Step 4. Data Gathering

The fourth element of the process calls for OHTA staff to define all alternative technologies for care of a clinical condition and to gather the data required for each objective priority-setting criterion.

Step 5. Creating Criterion Scores

In this step, a broadly representative subpanel would use consensus methods to create subjective criterion scores. A subpanel that included members with clinical experience and expertise in epidemiology and health statistics would determine criterion scores for objective criteria using data assembled for each clinical condition.

Step 6. Computing Priority Scores

The quantitative model developed by the committee and presented in Chapter 4 combines empirical rates (objective criterion scores) and subjective ratings (subjective criterion scores) as developed by the subpanels mentioned in step 5. Weighted criteria are multiplied by the natural logarithm of the criterion scores for each condition and technology and combined to form a single priority score for ranking.

Step 7. Review of Priority Rankings by the National Advisory Council of the Agency for Health Care Policy and Research

The AHCPR National Advisory Council would review the priority list and adjust it if desired before advising the AHCPR administrator to implement the set of priorities for assessment.

Resources for Implementation

The committee has carefully considered how best to implement the priority-setting process and to meet the requirements implementation may impose for additional resources while still achieving the goals of a credible, sound, defensible model process. This priority-setting process, based on the committee's experience with the pilot test, is likely to require more resources to respond to its expanded mission than are currently available. The committee thus viewed its work in part as a strategic effort to look ahead to reasonable goals for AHCPR and OHTA and to characterize the kinds and levels of program resources that would be needed.

The committee concluded that the importance of the priority-setting effort warrants a staff large enough to accomplish its mission of helping to use the country's technology assessment resources wisely. The committee believes implementing its process will require staffing at least comparable to that for a grant review study section. Human resources needed to implement the proposed process include program staff and priority-setting panels.

The Priority-Setting Cycle

Priority setting for OHTA should occur approximately every 3 years. The broadly representative panels that are constituted to carry it out have four tasks (described in steps 1, 3, and 5 above). Panel task 1, which is initially to select criteria and set criterion weights, occurs approximately once every 5 years; panel tasks 2 through 4 would occur about once every 3 years. These latter tasks are, respectively, to reduce the long list of candidate conditions and technologies to a more manageable size (i.e., "winnowing"), to generate subjective criterion scores, and to generate objective criterion scores.

Throughout the 3-year cycle, OHTA program staff would be responsible for tracking information related to previous assessments.

Publicly Available Products

The committee views the priority-setting process as a public good that will be one of OHTA's most valued products; thus, OHTA should generate a list of priorities for assessment that is extensive enough for use by other organizations that perform technology assessment. Of further benefit will be the data base that OHTA creates during the process of compiling data for the quantitative model. The data base (containing such information, for example, as cost per case of the top-ranked conditions) will itself be a resource to other organizations.

Topics with Insufficient Evidence for Assessment Based on Review of the Literature

The committee suggested three possible responses to lack of scientific comparative data for assessment of a condition or technology. For instance, assessors might prepare an interim statement that would estimate how effective the technology would have to be for it to be cost-effective. Alternatively, they might use decision modeling as an interim approach until sufficient data are available, or they might encourage primary research; they might also employ combinations of these steps. Topics that are of high priority for assessment and for which there is insufficient evidence should be identified and proposed as a topic for further research that might be encouraged and supported by AHCPR. This concept of linking priority setting, assessment of the evidence, and a research agenda is an important foundation for technology assessment and for evidence-based medical practice. Indeed, the committee recommends that AHCPR adopt this approach to setting its research agenda.

ADOPTION OF THE IOM'S PRIORITY-SETTING PROCESS BY OTHER ORGANIZATIONS

Many organizations evaluate health technology, although the major categories of such organizations are third-party payers, such as the Health Care Financing Administration (HCFA) and the Blue Cross and Blue Shield Association (BCBSA), and associations that represent physicians, such as the American College of Physicians (as described in Chapter 2). The committee developed this proposal for a priority-setting process with the expectation that the process would apply and be useful to these and similar organizations as well as to OHTA.

Requests from HCFA's Bureau of Policy Development at present constitute almost the entire workload of OHTA, but the bureau has no formal system for selecting technologies that are to be evaluated by OHTA. BCBSA member plans conduct their own technology evaluations, which are used, in part, to make coverage decisions. The member plans also rely on information supplied by the national BCBSA organization, which has an internal technology assessment program for new and emerging technologies and which has commissioned several major programs of assessment of established technologies by the American College of Physicians (ACP, 1990, 1991). The committee believes that most of its recommendations for a priority-setting process will apply to these private organizations as well as to OHTA, for the following reasons:

- Although these organizations are part of the private sector, they also constitute a major public resource, both individually and collectively. The more they structure their technology assessment activities, including priority setting, as a public service, the greater the good they will do for their own private purposes and for their mission of public service. By focusing on clinical conditions rather than on individual technologies, their assessments are more likely to compare relevant alternative patient care strategies.
- The argument that priorities for assessment should be determined on

the basis of several criteria is quite generalizable. An organization that uses only one dimension (e.g., cost, burden of illness) is oversimplifying a very complex matter. The trade-off between cost and effectiveness is one of the most important questions that physicians and patients must understand and resolve daily in the office or hospital. Those who pay for care and those who provide it will, ultimately, disadvantage themselves if they focus only on one dimension of health technology. The committee has maintained that the first objective of modeling is to develop a model that reflects the organization's mission, and it is entirely possible that a company's mission is primarily to increase shareholder value. In this instance, the firm arguably cannot be expected to place much emphasis on serving the national interest. Nevertheless, some on the committee take a broader view, believing that even for-profit concerns should, in their own long-term self-interest, adopt a "national interest" perspective as well. To the extent this proposition is true, groups that do not adopt a "multifactorial" approach to priority setting may short-change their own interests as well as those of the nation.

- Because the committee's process accommodates the choice of any priority-setting criteria, an organization may choose criteria that serve its own interests. The committee argues, however, that public trust, which sustains any large organization of payers or professionals, requires criteria that are responsive to the public interest, as exemplified by the committee's seven criteria.
- If one accepts the argument that any organization performing health technology assessment, or the officers of that organization who are responsible for the technology assessment, are accountable to the public, at least in very general terms, it would seem to follow that any process of establishing priority rankings should be open, explicit, and understandable. Although the priority-setting process could simply involve implicit judgments about how well a candidate topic meets explicit criteria, an explicit method for determining priority rankings is better than an implicit method at satisfying the requirement for openness.
- The process of soliciting nominations is one element of an ideal process that could be designed to satisfy the needs of a specific organization without compromising the public interest.
- The committee believes that any program of technology assessment must encompass a commitment to reassess topics that have been previously assessed. This commitment must be supported by a program to monitor previously assessed topics for new information that might prompt a reassessment. The rationale for this recommendation is public accountability, but it applies to private interests as well. For example, an organization of physicians should not have a potentially obsolete policy on the public record. Neither should a payer continue to provide or to withhold coverage

on the basis of information that may have been superseded by newly published data.

Technology Assessment and Clinical Practice Guidelines

The committee's priority-setting process may also be useful in setting priorities for developing practice guidelines. At present, many organizations, including AHCPR's Forum for Quality and Effectiveness in Health Care, actually produce practice guidelines or support their development. Clinical practice guidelines, according to another IOM committee's definition (IOM, 1990c), are "systematically developed statements to assist the practitioner and patient in decisions concerning appropriate health care for specific clinical circumstances." This and a forthcoming IOM report, *Guidelines for Clinical Practice: From Development to Use*, call attention to the following needs: information on costs and outcomes; a rigorous, open, and documented development process; a broadly representative, multidisciplinary process of development and review; and a systematic plan for scheduled review and reassessments.

Clinical practice guidelines are one vehicle for disseminating the results of technology assessment, and technology assessment is one method of producing information for a practice guideline. In particular, clinical practice guidelines may use the synthesis of available evidence and projection of outcomes that are a part of technology assessment as a foundation for statements that are clinically useful in individual patient care. Good practice guidelines go one step further, however, to rely on expert consensus to develop practical advice for clinicians in situations not directly addressed by clinical research.

What further distinguishes practice guidelines from technology assessment is the requirement that guidelines very carefully and explicitly describe the thinking that links the evidence (that is, the product of the technology assessment), or the lack of evidence, with the advice. Nonetheless, because technology assessment is so closely related to the development of practice guidelines, the priority-setting process proposed in this report appears to be largely, if not completely, applicable to guidelines development as well.

POTENTIAL PROBLEMS WITH THE PRIORITY-SETTING PROCESS

There are some potential problems with the process proposed in this report, but the committee believes that most of them stem from misperceptions about the use of a quantitative model to calculate a priority score. The great advantages of the model process are that it is explicit, that it contains a representation of the values of society, and that it defines the information-gathering tasks involved in setting priorities. Balanced against these advantages are three main concerns.

Will a Numerical Priority Score Lead to Unrealistic Inferences About Priority?

The output of the model will be a priority score that can be calculated to several decimal places if necessary. Although the model encourages precise thinking about the factors that are important in setting priorities, it is not (and cannot be) a more precise tool than the data used to estimate criterion scores. Several of the criterion scores are numerical representations of subjective judgments. The definitions of the criterion scores, as described in Chapter 4, are precise to encourage panelists to adopt the same set of assumptions when they make subjective judgments. But a criterion score is precise only if it has a small coefficient of variation across all panel members.

The risk of imputing false precision to a priority score is that it may lead to erroneous inferences that one of two candidates with similar (but not identical) priority scores has a stronger claim to priority because of its higher score. Nevertheless, the possibility that such a false judgment could occur is not a weakness of the priority-setting process. An organization might counteract such inferences by grouping candidates with similar scores and making choices among them, if need be, on the basis of other criteria (e.g., required timeliness or the expected cost of the assessment).

Does Codifying an Idealized Process Lead to Inflexibility?

This report has emphasized the way in which the proposed process can take into account the factors that should be important in deciding whether to assess a technology. Is there a risk that this process is too precise for the political climate of technology assessment? Does the system need more "give" than is provided by a quantitative model that generates a priority score? The committee argues, rather, that an explicit process facilitates open discussion. Furthermore, the rank-ordered list (or, if preferable, the groupings of candidate topics with similar scores) should be understood as no more than one kind of information to inform a political process by which to choose the final set of topics for technology assessment.

Will There Be a Bias Toward Choosing Topics That Are Quantifiable?

As Freymann (1974) has noted, "The Cartesian physician tended to forget that not everything we can count counts, nor can everything that counts be counted." To calculate a priority score, the proposed system requires data. Does this requirement mean that topics for which data are not available will be less likely to be assessed? Perhaps so, but a close look at the criteria suggests that this danger is more apparent than real.

First, four of the criteria do not require data. These subjective criteria require the panelist to make a subjective estimate and to express it on a scale of 1 to 5. Estimating a score for these criteria will not cause systematic bias against certain topics because the estimation problem will exist for all topics.

Second, of the remaining three criteria, one is the expected unit cost of the procedure for managing the condition; another is the prevalence of the condition. Analysts should be able either to collect or to estimate these data fairly easily.

The last criterion, the coefficient of variation of use rates, will be the most difficult in terms of data collection because it requires that the clinical condition or procedure be used on a wide enough scale to calculate meaningful use rates. The administrative data sets that many investigators study have a substantial advantage in the investigation of rare conditions because the largest ones can contain almost the entire population of such events in the United States. In the worst case—no available data on variation in use rates—the panel would simply assign the mean coefficient of variation of all other candidate topics.

CONCLUSION

Although this committee has recommended a specific step-by-step methodology as a priority-setting process, it believes that the four principles noted earlier in this report are far more important than the specifics of its model. First, the entire enterprise must be consistent with the mission of the organization. Second, the results of the process should be consistent with the needs of the user and should provide information in the form that is most useful. Third, the process should be efficient, especially in instances in which it must share resources with technology assessment itself. Fourth, the process must consider the political, economic, and social constraints that will affect how the information can be used. In the case of OHTA, satisfying the first principle will require determining which assessments are most likely to result in improvement in the health of the public, reduction of inappropriate health care expenditures, reduction of inequities in access to effective health care services or of maldistribution across equally needy populations, and the informing of other ethical, legal, and social issues.

OHTA and other organizations may wish to modify some of the components of the process as proposed. Experience with using this method or others will provide a sound basis for change, and organizations should constantly reexamine their methods for setting priorities. When making any changes, these groups should consider carefully whether modifying a given element might adversely affect the performance of the entire process.

In proposing a strategy for an optimal priority-setting process, the committee realizes that funding for technology assessment is already constrained and that its proposed priority-setting system will require some additional resources. Given the potential value of priority setting, however, the funding for this effort appears to be justified.

The committee views its report as a strategic effort to look ahead to reasonable goals for AHCPR and OHTA and to create a process that will be credible, sound, and defensible. During the process of compiling data for the quantitative model, OHTA will create a valuable data base and a ranking of priorities; both will be important resources for other organizations as well as for OHTA itself. Indeed, such a program could lead not only to wise use of public and private resources for technology assessment but also to an increase in public support for the entire technology assessment process.

References

ACP (American College of Physicians). *Common Diagnostic Tests: Use and Interpretation.* Sox, H.C., ed. Philadelphia, Pa.: The College, 1990.
ACP. *Common Screening Tests.* Eddy, D.M., ed. Philadelphia, Pa.: The College, 1991.
Altman, S.H., and Blendon, R., eds. *Medical Technology: The Culprit Behind Health Care Costs? Proceedings of the 1977 Sun Valley Forum on National Health* . Washington, D.C.: U.S. Government Printing Office, 1979. Publ. No. (PHS) 79-3216.
AMA (American Medical Association). *DATTA: Diagnostic and Therapeutic Technology Assessment.* Chicago, Ill.: AMA, 1988.
Banta, D.H., and Thacker, S.B. The Case for Reassessment of Health Care Technology. *Journal of the American Medical Association* 264:235-239, 1990.
Banta, D.H., Behney, C.J., and Williams, J.S. *Toward Rational Technology in Medicine.* New York: Springer, 1981.
Blumenthal, D. Federal Policy Toward Health Care Technology: The Case of the National Center. *Milbank Memorial Fund Quarterly* 61:584-613, 1983.
Brook, R.H., and Lohr, K.N. Will We Need to Ration Effective Health Care? *Issues in Science and Technology* 3:68-77, 1986.
Brown, L.D. The National Politics of Oregon's Rationing Plan. *Health Affairs* 10:29-51, Summer 1991.
Brown, R.E., Sheingold, S.H., and Luce, B.R. *Options of Using Practice Guidelines in Reducing the Volume of Medically Unnecessary Services* . BHARC-013/89/ 027. Washington, D.C.: Battelle Human Affairs Research Centers, 1989.
Callahan, D. Commentary: Ethics and Priority Setting in Oregon. *Health Affairs* 10:78-87, Summer 1991.
Chassin, M.R., Brook, R.H., Park, R.E., et al. Variations in the Use of Medical and Surgical Services by the Medicare Population. *New England Journal of Medicine* 314:285-290, 1986.

REFERENCES

Chassin, M.R., Kosecoff, J., Park, R.E., et al. Does Inappropriate Use Explain Geographic Variations in the Use of Health Care Services? A Study of Three Procedures. *Journal of the American Medical Association* 258:2533-2537, 1987.

Coile, R.C. Technology and Ethics: Three Scenarios for the 1990s. *Quality Review Bulletin* 16:202-208, 1990.

DHHS (Department of Health and Human Services). *AHCPR. Purpose and Programs.* Rockville, Md.: DHHS, September 1990. Publ. No. OM90-0096.

Eddy, D.M. Variations in Physician Practice: The Role of Uncertainty. *Health Affairs* 3:74-89, 1984.

Eddy, D.M. Selecting Technologies for Assessment. *International Journal of Technology Assessment in Health Care* 5:485-501, 1989.

Eddy, D.M. Designing a Practice Policy. Standards, Guidelines, and Options. *Journal of the American Medical Association* 263:3077-3084, 1990a.

Eddy, D.M. Guidelines for Policy Statements: The Explicit Approach. *Journal of the American Medical Association* 263:877-880, 1990b.

Eddy, D.M. Practice Policies—What Are They? *Journal of the American Medical Association* 263:1265-1275, 1990c.

Eddy, D.M., and Billings, J. The Quality of the Medical Evidence. *Health Affairs* 7:20-32, Spring 1988.

Ellwood, P.M. Outcomes Management: A Technology of Patient Experience. *New England Journal of Medicine* 318:1549-1556, 1988.

Etzioni, A. (Commentary) Health Care Rationing: A Critical Evaluation. *Health Affairs* 10:88-95, Summer 1991.

Fowler, P.J., Jr., Wennberg, J.E., Timothy, R.P., et al. Symptom Status and Quality of Life Following Prostatectomy. *Journal of the American Medical Association* 259:3018-3022, 1988.

Freymann, J. *The American Health Care System: Its Genesis and Trajectory*. New York: Medcom Press, 1974; quoted in Banta et al. (1981).

Fuchs, V.R., and Garber, A.M. The New Technology Assessment. *New England Journal of Medicine* 323:673-677, 1990.

Gelijns, A. Comparing the Development of Drugs, Devices, and Clinical Procedures. Pp. 147-201 in *Modern Methods of Clinical Investigations*, Vol. 1 in the series *Medical Innovation at the Crossroads*. Washington, D.C.: National Academy Press, 1990.

Gelijns, A., and Thief, S. Medical Technology Development: An Introduction to the Innovation-Evaluation Nexus. Pp. 1-15 in *Modern Methods of Clinical Investigation*, Vol. 1. in the series *Medical Innovation at the Crossroads*. Washington, D.C.: National Academy Press, 1990.

Ginsberg, E. High Tech Medicine and Rising Health Care Costs. *Journal of the American Medical Association* 263:1820-1822, 1990.

Holohan, J., Berenson, R.A., and Kachavos, P.G. Area Variations in Selected Medicare Procedures. *Health Affairs* 9:166-175, Winter 1990.

IOM (Institute of Medicine). *Assessing Medical Technologies*. Committee for Evaluating Medical Technologies in Clinical Use, Division of Health Sciences Policy, and Division of Health Promotion and Disease Prevention. Washington, D.C.: National Academy Press, 1985.

IOM. *Council on Health Care Technology, 1986-1987*. Washington, D.C.: National Academy Press, 1988.

IOM. *Effectiveness Initiative: Setting Priorities for Clinical Conditions.* Lohr, K.N., and Rettig, R.A., eds. Washington, D.C.: National Academy Press, 1989a.
IOM. *The NLM and Health Care Technology Assessment. Report of a Study by the Information Panel of the Council for Health Care Technology.* Washington, D.C.: National Academy Press, 1989b.
IOM. *Acute Myocardial Infarction: Setting Priorities for Effectiveness Research.* Mattingly, P.H., and Lohn:, K.N., eds. Washington, D.C.: National Academy Press, 1990a.
IOM. *Breast Cancer: Setting Priorities for Effectiveness Research.* Lohr, K.N., ed. Washington, D.C.: National Academy Press, 1990b.
IOM. *Clinical Practice Guidelines: Directions for a New Program.* Field, M.J., and Lohr, K.N., eds. Washington, D.C.: National Academy Press, 1990c.
IOM. *Effectiveness and Outcomes in Health Care.* Proceedings of an Invitational Conference by the Institute of Medicine. Heithoff, K.A., and Lohr, K.N., eds. Washington, D.C.: National Academy *Press*, 1990d.
IOM. *Hip Fracture: Setting Priorities for Effectiveness Research.* Lohr, K.N., and Heithoff, K.A., eds. Washington, D.C.: National Academy Press, 1990e.
IOM. *National Priorities for the Assessment of Clinical Conditions and Medical Technologies: Report of a Pilot Study.* Lara, M.E., and Goodman, C., eds. Washington, D.C.: National Academy Press, 1990f.
IOM. *The Computer-Based Patient Record. An Essential Technology for Health Care.* Dick, R., and Steen, E.B., eds. Washington, D.C.: National Academy Press, 1991a.
IOM. *Improving Information Services for Health Services Researchers.* A Report to the National Library of Medicine. Harris-Wehling, J., and Morris, L.C., eds. Washington, D.C.: The Institute, 1991b.
IOM. *Guidelines for Clinical Practice: From Development to Use.* Field, M.J., and Lohr, K.N., eds. Washington, D.C.: National Academy *Press*, forthcoming.
Kinney, E.D. Report to the Administrative Conference of the United States on National Coverage Policy Under the Medicare Program: Problems and Proposals for Change. The Center for Law and Health, Indiana University School of Law, November 1987.
Kuppermann, M., Luce, B.R., McGovern, B., et al. An Analysis of the Cost-Effectiveness of the Implantable Cardiac Defibrillator. *Circulation* 81:91-100, 1990.
Leaf, A. Cost Effectiveness as a Criterion for Medicare Coverage. *New England Journal of Medicine* 321:898-900, 1989.
Lewin and Associates. *A Forward Plan for Medicare Coverage and Technology Assessment.* Vol. 1: The Forward Plan. Roe, W., Anderson, M., Gong, I., et al., eds. Washington, D.C.: Lewin and Associates, 1987.
Lohr, K.N. Outcome Measurement: Concepts and Questions. *Inquiry* 25:37-50, 1988.
McNeil, B.J., and Abrams, H.L. *Brigham and Women's Handbook of Diagnostic Imaging.* Boston, Mass.: Little, Brown, 1986.
McNeil, B.J., Weichselbaum, R., and Pauker, S.G. Fallacy of the Five-year Survival in Lung Cancer. *New England Journal of Medicine* 299:1397-1401, 1978.
McPhee, S.J., Myers, L.P., and Schroeder, S.A. The Cost and Risks of Medical

Care—An Annotated Bibliography for Clinicians and Educators. *Western Journal of Medicine* 137:145-161, 1982.

McPherson, K., Wennberg, J.E., Hovind, O.B., et al. Small Area Variations in the Use of Common Surgical Procedures: An International Comparison of New England, England, and Norway. *New England Journal of Medicine* 307:1310-1314, 1982.

Merrick, N.L., Brook, R.H., link, A., et al. Use of Carotid Endarterectomy in Five California Veterans Administration Medical Centers. *Journal of the American Medical Association* 258:2531-2535, 1986.

Misener, J.H. The Impact of Technology on the Quality of Health Care. *Quality Review Bulletin* 16:209-213, June 1990.

Moloney, T.W., and Rogers, D.E. Medical Technology—A Different View of the Continuous Debate over Costs. *New England Journal of Medicine* 301:1413-1419, 1979.

Moskowitz, A.J., Benjamin, J.K., and Kassirer, J.P. Dealing with Uncertainty, Risks, and Tradeoffs in Clinical Decisions . *Annals of Internal Medicine* 108:435-449, 1988.

Mushlin, A.I. Uncertain Decisionmaking in Primary Care: Causes and Solutions. Pp. 153-158 in *Primary Care Research: Theory and Methods*. Rockville, Md.: DHHS, 1991. Publ. No. 91-0011.

National Advisory Council on Health Care Technology Assessment. The Medicare Coverage Process. Submitted to the Secretary of Health and Human Services and the Director of the National Center for Health Services Research and Health Care Technology Assessment. September 1988.

Office of Inspector General. *Medicare Carrier Assessment of New Technologies*. Washington, D.C.: DHHS, April 1990. Publ. No. OEI-01-88-00010.

OTA (Office of Technology Assessment). *Assessing the Efficacy and Safety of Medical Technologies*. U.S. Congress. Washington, D.C.: U.S. Government Printing Office, 1978. Publ. No. OTA-H-75.

OTA. *The Implications of Cost-Effectiveness Analysis of Medical Technology*. Background Paper No. 1: Methodological Issues and Literature Review. U.S. Congress. Washington, D.C.: U.S. Government Printing Office, 1980.

OTA. *Strategies for Medical Technology Assessment*. U.S. Congress. Washington, D.C.: U.S. Government Printing Office, 1982.

Park, R.E., Fink, A., Brook, R.H., et al. *Physician Ratings of Appropriate Indications for Six Medical and Surgical Procedures* . R-3280-CWF/HF/PMT/RWJ. Santa Monica, Calif.: The RAND Corporation, 1986.

Paul-Shaheen, P., Clark, J.D., and Williams, D. Small Area Analysis: A Review and Analysis of the North American Literature. *Journal of Health Politics, Policy and Law* 12:741-809, 1987.

Perry, S., and Pillar, B. A National Policy for Health Care Technology Assessment (editorial). *Medical Care Review* 47:401-416, 1990.

Phelps, C.E. Death and Taxes—An Opportunity for Substitution. *Journal of Health Economics* 7:1-24, 1988.

Phelps, C.E. Diffusion of Information in Medical Care. *Journal of Economic Perspectives*. Forthcoming.

Phelps, C.E., and Mooney, K. Variation in Medical Practice Use: Causes and Consequences. University of Rochester, June 1991.

Phelps, C.E., and Parente, S.T. Priority Setting in Medical Technology and Medical Practice Assessment. *Medical Care* 28:703-723, 1990.
Relman, A.S. Assessment and Accountability: The Third Revolution in Medical Care. *New England Journal of Medicine* 319:1220-1222, 1988.
Rettig, R.A. Technology Assessment—An Update. *Investigative Radiology* 26:165-173, 1991.
Roberts, E.B. Technological Innovation and Medical Devices. Pp. 35-47 in *New Medical Devices*. Ekelman, K.B., ed. Washington, D.C.: National Academy Press, 1988.
Roper, W.L., Winkenwerder, W., Hackbarth, G.M., et al. Effectiveness in Health Care: An Initiative to Evaluate and Improve Medical Practice. *New England Journal of Medicine* 319:1197-1202, 1988.
Schwartz, W.B. The Inevitable Failure of Cost Containment Strategies. *Journal of the American Medical Association* 257:220-224, 1987.
Sipes-Metzler, P.R. Oregon's Challenge to Achieve Health Care Equity. Paper presented at a meeting sponsored by the California Public Employees' Retirement System's Health Benefits Advisory Council, April 24-25, 1991.
Snedecor, G.W., and Cochran, W.G. *Statistical Methods*. Ames, Iowa: The Iowa State University Press, 1967.
Stewart, A.L., Greenfield, S., Hays, R.D., et al. Functional Status and Well-being of Patients With Chronic Conditions. Results from the Medical Outcomes Study. *Journal of the American Medical Association* 262:907-913, 1989.
Wells, K.B., Stewart, A., and Hays, R.D. The Functioning and Well-being of Depressed Patients. Results from the Medical Outcomes Study. *Journal of the American Medical Association* 262:914-919, 1989.
Wennberg, J.E. The Paradox of Appropriate Care. *Journal of the American Medical Association* 258:2568-2569, 1987.
Wennberg, J.E. What is Outcomes Research? Pp. 33-46 in *Modern Methods of Clinical Investigation*, Vol. 1 in the series *Medical Innovation at the Crossroads*. Washington, D.C.: National Academy Press, 1990.
Wennberg, J.E., and Gittelsohn, A. Small Area Variations in Health Care Delivery. *Science* 142:1102-1108, 1973.
Wennberg, J.E., and Gittelsohn, A. Health Care Delivery in Maine. I: Patterns of Use of Common Surgical Procedures. *Journal of the Maine Medical Association* 66:123-149, 1975.
Wennberg, J.E., and Gittelsohn, A. Variations in Medical Care Among Small Areas. *Scientific American* 246:120-134, 1982.
Winslow, C.M., Solomon, D.H., Chassin, M.R., et al. The Appropriateness of Carotid Endarterectomy. *New England Journal of Medicine* 318:721-727, 1988a.
Winslow, C.M., Kosecoff, J.B., Chassin, M.R., et al. The Appropriateness of Performing Coronary Artery Bypass Surgery. *Journal of the American Medical Association* 260:505-509, 1988b.
Woolf, S.H., Battista, R.N., Anderson, O.M., et al. Assessing the Clinical Effectiveness of Preventive Maneuvers: Analytic Principles and Systematic Methods in Reviewing Evidence and Developing Clinical Practice Recommendations. The Canadian Task Force on the Periodic Health Examination. *Journal of Clinical Epidemiology* 43:891-905, 1990.

Appendix A
Pilot Test of the IOM Model

In July 1991, five members of the Committee on Priorities for Health Technology Assessment and Reassessment convened to pilot-test the committee's model for priority setting. The version they tested was designated the convened pilot; a second mailed pilot test provided clam for a comparison of the results obtained by each method, convening and mailing. The purpose of the pilot testing was (1) to test the methodology, (2) to compare results of the two groups to judge whether a mail process was a reasonable substitute for a convened group, and (3) to use the experience of both groups to improve the model.

Each group used a consensus process to assign weights to the six criteria that the full committee had chosen at an earlier meeting; group members also assigned criterion scores by vote for the three subjective criteria (a seventh criterion was later added by the committee). In addition, the convened group estimated missing data where needed to assign criterion scores for objective data. The mailed pilot test used the criterion definitions developed by the convened group to weight the criteria and provided criterion scores for the three subjective criteria.

In addition to the weighting and criterion scoring activities, each group listed the ethical, legal, and social problems that contributed to their rating of that criterion. This report compares the products of both groups and draws conclusions about implementation of the model.

METHODS

Topics and Data for Priority Setting

To prepare for the pilot test, study staff sampled 11 conditions and technologies from a rank-ordered list of 20 topics produced during the IOM/CHCT pilot study (IOM, 1990f). Using stratified random sampling, the first- and twentieth-ranked conditions or technologies were sampled first. Nine additional topics were then sampled between the top and bottom of the group using a table of random numbers.

Conditions and technologies were defined more specifically than in the IOM/CHCT study to facilitate data gathering. These definitions required a designation of whether the condition or technology was to include prevention, screening, diagnosis, or treatment; the level of severity; the care settings; and the anatomical site or sites of interest. For instance, "cardiovascular disease" in the IOM/CHCT study was further defined for this pilot test as "treatment of coronary artery disease severe enough to consider revascularization but not treatment of post-myocardial infarction." Thus, the individual topics in the pilot test were a subset of the topics listed in the IOM/CHCT report but not strictly comparable to them.

Before the meeting, staff compiled data on each condition and technology and provided the pilot-test group with a summary describing each condition, a list of alternative technologies to be considered, and data relevant to each condition.

Although the groups were small (each had six members), they included clinicians and individuals experienced in quantitative and health services research and technology assessment, and public policymaking.

Criteria

The following six criteria were to be weighted and given criterion scores:

1. burden of illness (per patient with the disease)
2. cost (expenditures/person/year)
3. prevalence (rate/1,000 in the general population)
4. practice variations (coefficient of variation)
5. potential of the assessment to improve health outcomes
6. potential of the assessment to resolve ethical, legal, or social (ELS) issues.

Mailed pilot-test respondents were given instructions about how to assign weights and subjective scores for each criterion. After the pilot test was completed, the committee further refined the definitions of each criterion (see Chapter 4).

Criterion Weighting

The pilot group voted to take one criterion—the ELS criterion, which in some respects was considered the least important—and use it to anchor the bottom end of the weighting scale. Each member of the group then assigned weights to the remaining five criteria relative to his or her perception of the importance of the rating of ELS ("How much more important is criterion X than ELS?"). The group discussed individual weights and voted again. The mean weights that were computed following this round were used for the remainder of the pilot test. The mailed pilot test group had only one round of voting.

Criterion Scoring

Convened Pilot

Objective Criterion Scores.

The group reviewed the data that the staff had assembled and discussed which data were pertinent to the criteria. After ensuring that measures were used consistently among conditions and technologies, the group estimated missing data for the three objective criteria—prevalence, costs, and practice variations.

Subjective Criterion Scores. Each member of the convened pilot group independently rated the conditions and technologies on burden of illness, potential to improve outcomes, and potential to resolve ELS issues. The group then discussed their scores and had an opportunity to make adjustments (such adjustment occurred in 27 of 135 separate ratings for the convened group). The ratings for each condition, as would be expected, showed regression to the mean. Mean scores for each criterion were entered in the quantitative model to calculate priority scores.

Mailed Pilot

Objective Criterion Scores. The mailed pilot test group was not asked to provide objective criterion scores. Consequently, in order to compare priority scores for both groups, the analysis used the criterion scores that the convened pilot group assigned to each criterion (as well as the convened pilot criterion weights) to compute priority scores for both groups on the objective criteria.

Subjective Criterion Scores. Members of both groups rated each of the three subjective criteria based on summary descriptive material about each condition and technology and available data on burden of illness. Each respondent indicated the reasoning behind his or her rating for ELS issues.

RESULTS

Feasibility

The convened group concluded that its model was feasible. Staff time required to assemble data for each condition was approximately 1 day. Although many data were missing or expressed in noncomparable units, the group found that the criteria could be operationally defined and that its combined experience was sufficient to estimate data (although with the understanding that a full implementation of the model would require more complete data).

Improvements in the Model

Pilot testing led the committee to extensive deliberation about the criterion definitions and their appropriate units, and to the addition of one criterion, for a total of seven. The committee also considered and further clarified the composition of the panels for weighting the criteria and for creating subjective and objective criterion scores.

Comparison of Convened and Mailed Methods

Three questions might be asked about the two methods. First, how much dispersion was there around the mean for each group (within-group differences)? Second, how much did criterion scores differ when developed by a group process or by an individualized mail process without feedback (between-group differences)? Third, how much do differences in subjective scores contribute to differences in priority scores?

Criterion Weights

The first analysis addressed the differences between the two pilots in mean criterion weights and their dispersion. Figure A.1 shows the mean criterion weights and their standard deviations for the six members of the convened pilot group. Figure A.2 shows the mean criterion weights and standard deviations derived by the mailed pilot group. Overall, the mailed pilot group assigned higher individual criterion weights and had a greater range of weights relative to the ELS criterion than were assigned by the convened group. Within the mailed group, the highest ranking criterion—likelihood of an assessment changing health outcomes—reached a mean rating of 3.7; the highest weight assigned by the convened group was only 2.25 for burden of illness.

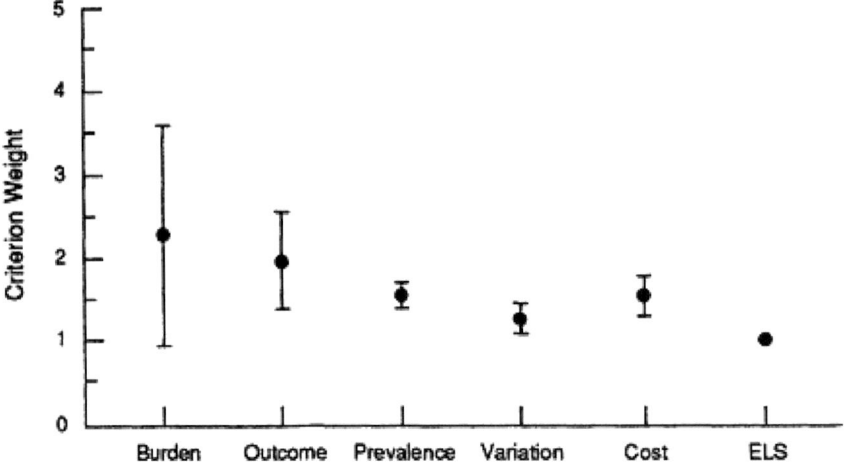

Figure A.1 Mean criterion weights and their standard deviations for the convened pilot group; ELS=ethical, legal, and social (issues).

Criterion Scores

Between-Group Comparisons. Criterion scores for the three subjective criteria (burden of illness, likelihood of an assessment changing health outcomes, and probability of resolving an ELS issue) were compared for each condition or technology. Overall, the mailed pilot group rated conditions higher (22 of 33 conditions were rated higher by the mailed pilot), although a sign test was not significant ($X^2 = 3.67$; Snedecor and Cochran, 1967).

Within-Group Dispersion of Responses. Standard deviations for each criterion score were also compared using a sign test. Here, the findings are striking, if not predictable. In 26 of 33 possible ratings, the standard deviations for the mailed group are larger, in many cases considerably larger, than for the convened group. Using the sign test to compare the number of condition and technology pairs in which one or the other group had a higher deviation in their ratings yields $X^2 = 10.93$ ($p <<.001$).

Taken together, the two sign tests indicated that despite small numbers of respondents (six in each group), the mailed pilot group had a significantly greater dispersion in responses, compared with the convened group, and rated each condition higher for most criteria.

Priority Scores

Observed Priority Scores (seeFigure A.3). For the objective criteria, the mailed pilot used the criterion weights and objective criterion scores derived by the convened pilot group. Thus, the two groups differ only on the subjective ratings. As in the assigning of criterion weights, the priority scores of the mailed pilot group were higher than those of the convened group for each condition. Relative priority scores for the two groups, however, were comparable. As can be seen in Figure A.3, scores for the top three conditions or technologies were approximately the same, as were scores for the bottom four.

Sensitivity of Priority Scores to Changes in Subjective Criterion Scores. The second analysis addressed the effect of a change in the subjective ratings on the resulting priority score. Given that the mailed pilot yielded greater variations in response, what effect do these variations have on the final priority score?

It is useful to examine how the model behaves when criterion scores vary (Figure A.4). To test how changes in subjective ratings affect the final priority score, one can hold constant the criterion weights and the objective

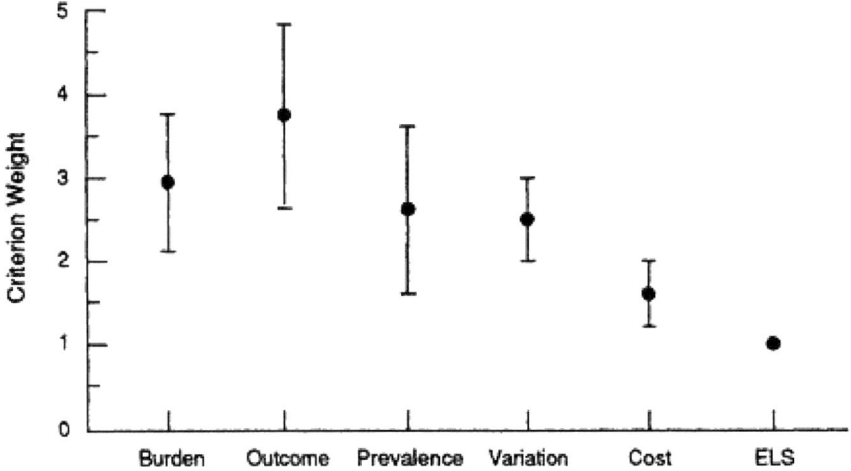

Figure A.2 Mean criterion weights and their standard deviations for the mailed pilot group; ELS=ethical, legal, and social (issues).

APPENDIX A

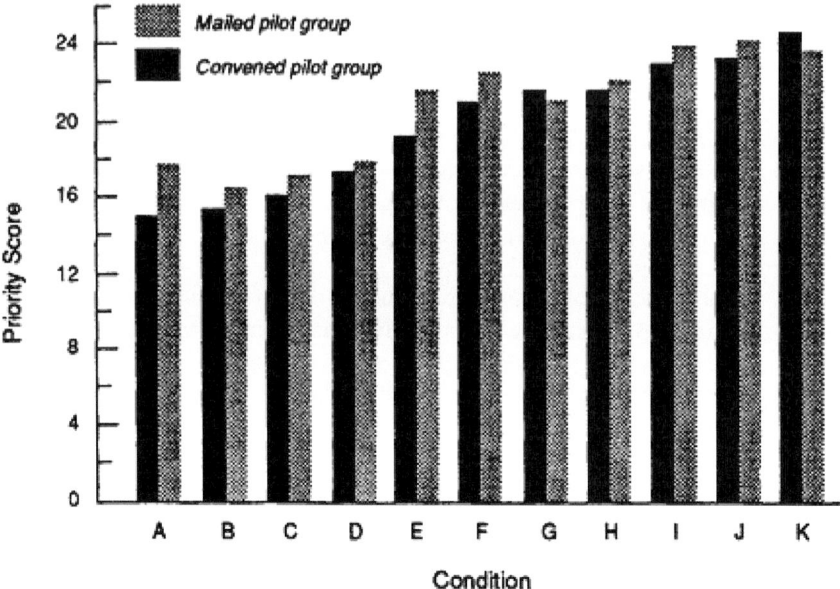

Figure A.3 Priority scores for the convened and mailed pilot groups.

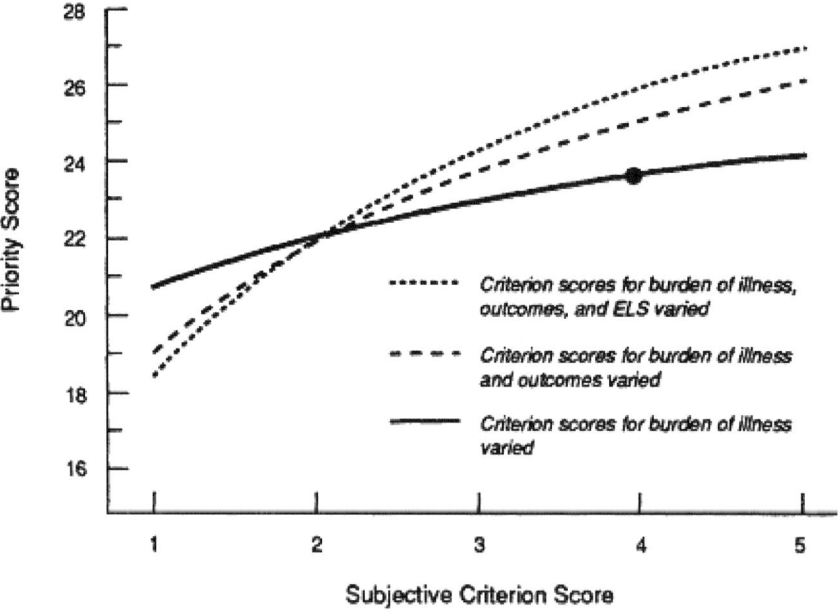

Figure A.4 Effect of varying the subjective criterion scores on the priority score; ELS=ethical, legal, and social (issues). The example used is a debilitating chronic illness.

criterion scores and vary first one, then two, and finally all three subjective ratings from their minimum to maximum values.

The solid circle in Figure A.4 shows the observed priority score of 23.6 for a debilitating chronic condition for which burden of illness was rated 4, outcomes 2, and ELS 1.9. The overlying curve shows the effect on the priority score when the rating for burden of illness is changed to 1, 2, 3, and 5.

The second curve (the dashed line) shows the result of varying two subjective ratings simultaneously; the third curve (the dotted line) shows the result of varying all three ratings. When all three ratings are varied from 1 to 5, the expected priority scores range from 18.45 to 26.9, which is equivalent to the 8.5-point range observed in this exercise for all the conditions considered (15.7-24.2). From this, one may draw conclusions about how the quantitative model behaves: although priority scores are robust (e.g., resistant to change caused by extremes in individual ratings), substantial changes in the mean criterion score for a given condition affect the final priority score.

IMPLICATIONS OF THE PILOT TESTS FOR THE IOM MODEL

Neither group reported difficulties in assigning criterion weights, although the group surveyed by mail reported difficulty in assigning subjective criterion scores for individual conditions or technologies. They attributed their difficulties to uncertainty about applying the criteria to specific conditions as well as about the scope of the technologies to include. Other problematic factors were incomplete data, some instances of data that were not expressed in comparable units, and lack of familiarity with a given clinical condition.

Criterion weights assigned by the convened group showed less dispersion (particularly after group discussion) than did those assigned by the mailed pilot group. Although members of the mailed pilot group received revised definitions of each criterion, the definitions were briefly stated and did not include applied examples. Individual mailed pilot criterion scores varied more widely and tended to be higher than the scores of the convened pilot group. The greater variation in response is easily explained by lack of group consensus about the meaning of the criteria or a chance to discuss and vote again, but it is not clear why the scores of the mailed pilot group tended to be higher. Despite these differences, and perhaps of greater interest, both groups rated burden of illness and outcome high relative to the other criteria. They also rated prevalence, practice variations, and cost above ELS issues.

Criterion Scores

The convened group derived objective criterion scores using a combination of the data provided by staff and their expertise and knowledge of the clinical conditions. The group needed to perform less estimation for prevalence and clinical practice variations than for costs. It should be noted that estimates of burden of illness must, at this time, be largely subjective. Although mortality data are readily available, health status measures that include functional status scores for a given clinical condition are still quite sparse in the clinical literature and require both clinical familiarity and patient- and family-based information.

Both the convened group and the mailed pilot group assigned scores to subjective criteria. Following the first round of ratings, the convened group used a Delphi process that focused on outlier ratings, differences in their interpretation of a criterion, and different features of the condition, patient populations, or social issues that each person had considered. In particular, ELS issues identified by group members varied widely.

For example, in explaining a high rating for the ELS criterion on cardiovascular procedures, one person cited the published differences in procedure rates for blacks and whites and what this implied about inequality of access. Another individual, who gave a rating of I to ELS issues, explained, "I seriously doubt new technology is as important as prevention." In considering the burden of illness from cataracts, one person persuaded the group that untreated cataracts could mean the difference between living independently and requiring nursing home care. Another person considered the burden to society of highway accidents related to cataract-impaired drivers. Considerations of treatment of alcoholism raised many social issues—for example, fetal alcohol syndrome, special at-risk populations, co-addiction, and issues related to insurance coverage for risky behavior. In considering intensive care units (ICUs), one member of the group focused on identifying the appropriate populations for ICU care, another on the implications of life-sustaining therapy for the terminally ill. In another example, considerations related to depression included underdiagnosis, depression associated with unemployment, the rising rate of teenage suicide, and side effects of medications. In some cases, the panel agreed that the issue was interesting but not relevant to setting priorities for technology assessment; in other cases, scores were adjusted as a result of the discussion.

The mailed pilot group, which did not have a second round of ratings, reported much more difficulty than the convened group in assigning ratings; the mailed group also had many more missing ratings. Respondents cited, in particular, lack of familiarity with the clinical condition and difficulty in understanding how to apply the criteria. One possible reason for the difference between the two groups is that the convening process gave individuals more confidence in assigning ratings (although not necessarily greater accuracy) in the face of almost complete uncertainty.

Although the number of individuals in each group was small, the two pilot tests suggest that implementation of the model will require very clear and careful descriptions of the criteria as well as several rounds of voting and discussion conducted in conference or by other methods to establish criterion weights. Some criteria, such as prevalence, are familiar to many people but are used in this model in specific ways, particularly when referring to procedures and screening technologies. Other criteria, such as burden of illness, are unfamiliar and require a clear definition to ensure that group members use them comparably.

The committee drew several conclusions from its pilot tests. First, the model is feasible, but those implementing it will need to establish a method (e.g., a training session or other form of education) to ensure a common understanding of the criteria. Second, there is considerable merit to using a two-stage group method that first anchors the ends of a given subjective criterion for a given candidate list and then assigns scores within these extremes. Third, it will be critical to establish the reliability of the criterion weighting process to ensure that the process is informed and stable—as well as efficient. Fourth, the model should be modified on the basis of use and experience. Aspects of validity include the reasonableness of the product and its acceptability to and employment by intended users. The committee's pilot test began this process of evaluation and modification, but it must be continued by the model's users.

Appendix B
Abbreviations

AHCPR	Agency for Health Care Policy and Research
BPD	Bureau of Policy Development
CHCT	Council on Health Care Technology
DHHS	Department of Health and Human Services
FDA	Food and Drug Administration
HCFA	Health Care Financing Administration
IOM	Institute of Medicine
NCHCT	National Center for Health Care Technology
NCHSR	National Center for Health Services Research and Health Care Technology Assessment
NIH	National Institutes of Health
OHTA	Office of Health Technology Assessment
OIG	Office of Inspector General
OTA	Office of Technology Assessment
PHS	Public Health Service